TOXIC OVERLOAD

The Invisible Endocrine-Disrupting Chemicals Making Us **SICK, FAT,** and **TIRED**

Evidence-Based Approaches to Overcome Health Issues in a Toxic World

S. M. René, MD, FACE, The EDC Doc™

Toxic Overload: The Invisible Endocrine-Disrupting Chemicals Making Us Sick, Fat, and Tired

Copyright © 2025 by S. M. René

All rights reserved. No part of this publication may be reproduced, distributed, or transmitted in any form or by any means, including photocopying, recording, or other electronic or mechanical methods, without the prior written permission of the copyright holder, except in the case of brief quotations embodied in critical reviews and certain other noncommercial uses permitted by copyright law.

Print ISBN: 979-8-218-83194-3
E-Book ISBN: 979-8-218-83195-0

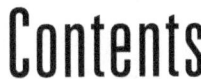

Contents

Introduction vii
How to Use This Book ix

Part One: Understand Your Enemy 1
Chapter One:
 Understanding Hormones and the Endocrine System 3
Chapter Two: What the Heck Are Endocrine-Disrupting
 Chemicals (EDCs)? 27
Chapter Three: Comprehending the Impact of EDCs and
 Their Link to Various Illnesses and Health Conditions 35
Chapter Four: How EDCs Are Making Us Sick:
 The Effects of EDCs on Health 39
Chapter Five: EDCs and Development of Prediabetes and
 Type 2 Diabetes 65
Chapter Six: The Relationship Between EDCs and the
 Development of Thyroid Disease 75
Chapter Seven: How EDCs Are Making Us Fat:
 Their Role as Obesogens. 79

Chapter Eight: How EDCs Are Making Us Tired:
  The Role of EDCs in Fatigue and Energy Levels. 121
Chapter Nine: Impacts of EDCs on Children and Adolescents . .131

**Part Two: This Is War! Strategies for Battling EDCs and
  Reclaiming Health** 135
Chapter Ten: Repairing the Liver:
  A Key Organ in Detoxification. 137
Chapter Eleven: Healing the Gut: Restoring Gut Health to
  Combat EDC Effects 147
Chapter Twelve: Go Green with Clean Food as Medicine: Optimal
  Nutrition to Counteract EDCs 155
Chapter Thirteen: How to Reduce Obesogens Naturally. 169
Chapter Fourteen: No More Plastics! Reducing Plastic Use to
  Minimize Exposure to EDCs in Everyday Life 183
Chapter Fifteen: A Breath of Fresh Air: How to Reduce Indoor
  and Outdoor Pollutants 187
Chapter Sixteen: Spring Cleaning Anytime: Using Safe Household
  Products and Eliminating EDC-Laden Products 191
Chapter Seventeen: Self-Care for Your Body: Choosing Clean
  Personal Care Products. 195
Chapter Eighteen: Relax, Relate, and Release! Emphasizing
  Relaxation and Stress Management for Overall Well-Being. . .199
Chapter Nineteen: Implementing the Battle on a Budget:
  Cost-Effective Approaches to Reducing EDC Exposures . . .211

**Part Three: Winning the War! Exploring Alternative Approaches
  to Reach Your Goal.** 215
Chapter Twenty: Chinese Medicine Perspective on Combating
  EDC Effects 217
Chapter Twenty-One: Ayurveda's Holistic Approach to Mitigating
  EDC Impact 221

Chapter Twenty-Two: Naturopathic Remedies and
   Recommendations Against EDCs. .227
Chapter Twenty-Three: Utilizing Essential Oils for Detoxification
   and Wellness 231
Chapter Twenty-Four: Vibrational Therapy to Promote
   Detoxification 235
Chapter Twenty-Five: To Detox or Not to Detox? Understanding
   the Pros and Cons of Detoxification Practices. 239
Chapter Twenty-Six: My Personal Journey 247
Chapter Twenty-Seven: Final Thoughts: Encouraging Ongoing
   Awareness and Action. 263

Glossary 267
Common Myths and Misconceptions 273
Frequently Asked Questions. 277
References. 285
List of Suggested Readings. 315
Recommended Resources. 317
Acknowledgments. 319
About the Author 321

Introduction

Over the past twenty-five years, I have been a practicing endocrinologist treating various conditions such as diabetes and thyroid, adrenal, and pituitary disorders, to name a few. In recent years, I have been challenged with increasing complaints from patients about persistent fatigue, weight gain, hair loss, and mood changes. I have also seen an increase in the incidence of diabetes and thyroid cancer cases. The standard recommendations taught in medical school to reduce caloric intake, increase exercise activity, and maintain a low-carb diet were no longer working. I kept seeing patients struggle despite all efforts to faithfully follow my recommendations. Then, at the age of forty-eight, I, too, became a victim of the same struggles. I was getting sick from frequent viral illnesses and was diagnosed with high blood pressure, prediabetes, and fatty liver disease. I later developed sleep apnea with persistent exhaustion. Many of these health problems were due to my creeping weight gain. My breaking point happened during a routine office visit with a patient whom I had not seen in two years. In the middle of our discussion, he remarked, "Hey, doc! I noticed you have gained a bit since I last saw you. You alright?" with his hands motioning to my midsection. Oh, the embarrassment and the anger I felt at that very moment. I kindly responded, "No, I'm OK. Thanks for asking. Let's get back to your diabetes." Was this a rude and inappropriate question? Absolutely! Was this my aha moment? Right again. This was the push I needed to compel me to do the research for answers and solutions, not only for myself but also for my struggling patients. Enough was enough! I subsequently came across a scientific article describing how toxins were hiding in our bodies' fat cells and leading to stubborn fat and difficulty with weight loss. Wait … what? Toxins stored in our fat cells? The proverbial light bulb came on. It is no wonder why so many of us are struggling to lose weight.

However, to make matters even worse, I later faced the dreaded "C" diagnosis. I developed blood and protein in my urine, along with stomach pains. A CT scan found a small, suspicious tumor in my right kidney with a 85 to 90 percent likelihood for renal cell carcinoma. This was a major shock, and it invigorated my quest to find out what environmental factors were contributing to my decline in health. You can read my full story and results in chapter twenty-six. Thus began my path to seek and share what I have learned with as many people as possible. I am here to tell everyone: *it's not your fault!* Toxins everywhere are overloading our bodies, leading to poor health and reduced wellness. Fortunately, hope is not lost. We now have ways to battle these invisible threats and invaders. I pray that you find this information enlightening, useful, and transformative, as it has been for me.

How to Use This Book

There are numerous expert opinions on how endocrine-disrupting chemicals (EDCs) cause autoimmune disorders, developmental problems, and even cancer. However, I intend to focus on how they affect our hormones, which in turn leads to countless diseases. Throughout this book, I will be sharing information about the different hostile forces waging war upon our bodies. I have included several QR codes for you to scan with your smartphone camera that will then take you to videos to help enhance your educational experience. Much like you'll see when using the free version of the Pandora app which has commercial ads, so, too, will you see the occasional ad pop up when you scan one of the included QR codes. There is no obligation to see the ad. Scan the QR code with your phone camera app. Click on the yellow link that pops up. Tap on the arrow for the video. Tap on "Close" to remove the ad. Then click on the arrow to play the video.

All videos are provided courtesy of Alilia Medical Media. Copying and/or downloading of any of the videos or animations to any social media platforms such as YouTube, Facebook, or TikTok is strictly prohibited.

The enemy is not just sugar but also these toxins that are wreaking havoc on our endocrine systems and hormones. I will outline science-based strategies to battle these enemy forces. With full disclosure, this is not a quick weight loss book or an instant healing program. The exposures to endocrine-disrupting chemicals occur through an insidious and prolonged process. So, too, will be the prevention, eradication, and recovery processes which will require determination and patience. Wars are not won in one day. With every step taken to reduce your exposure, you win the battle toward the ultimate victory for improved health and wellness.

Before starting any new diet, taking supplements, or making significant changes to your lifestyle, it is important to consult with your health-care provider. The information and advice provided in this book are not intended to replace professional medical consultation, diagnosis, or treatment. Your doctor can provide personalized advice based on your health history and current medical condition to ensure any new dietary changes or supplements are safe and appropriate for you.

As you delve deeper, you may find the information overwhelming and at times difficult to grasp fully. The reason for including such comprehensive data is not only to increase knowledge within the general public, but also to share with and educate my medical colleagues. My ultimate goal is to spark enough change to revolutionize how we approach chronic illnesses. Hopefully, one day in the near future, screening for toxins will become part of routine exams. I recommend taking a few small steps at a time as you move toward change. I have also included additional literature, resources, and websites to expand on what is gathered in this book. Just remember that you are not alone. This is war! This fight needs all of us— patients, doctors, wellness experts, scientists, politicians, and companies—to work together toward solutions that can be profitable for the industries while safeguarding our health. Ready to go to battle?

PART ONE:

Understand Your Enemy

CHAPTER ONE:

Understanding Hormones and the Endocrine System

To truly grasp the impact of endocrine-disrupting chemicals (EDCs) on our well-being, it's vital to first understand the intricate dance between hormones and their control tower: the endocrine system. Whenever I say hormones, most readers will immediately think of the female hormone estrogen and the male hormone testosterone. However, you may be surprised to know that the body makes over fifty different hormones. These hormones regulate various bodily functions from metabolism to growth. This chapter will be a comprehensive overview with a focus on the major hormones. This will serve as your guided tour through the complex but captivating world of hormones: what they are, what they do, and how they interact in a delicate balancing act to keep you healthy.

Think of hormones as the composers of a biological symphony. These potent chemical messengers, generated by various glands peppered throughout our bodies, are responsible for fine-tuning a host of essential bodily functions. Hormones circulate in your bloodstream seeking out specific cells which listen and respond to specific notes.

Once they find their target, they bind to specialized receptors on these cells, setting off a chain reaction of biological events. Another way to visualize this intricate system is to think of the hormone as a key and the receptor as a lock. The hormone unlocks the receptor to produce and release the hormone messengers toward their target organs for a desired metabolic effect.

Endocrine System

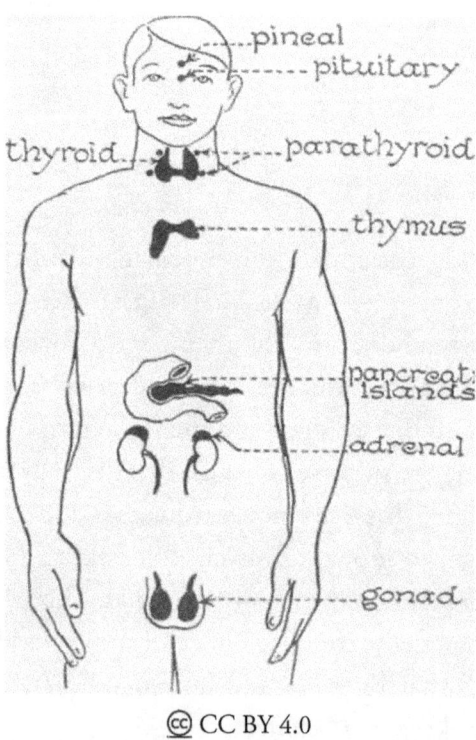

CC BY 4.0

The Endocrine Orchestra: Meet the Maestros

Picture the endocrine system as an orchestra, complete with a range of instruments—or, in this case, glands—each with its own distinct role in the production and delivery of hormones. The endocrine system is a network of glands throughout the body that produce hormones, chemical messengers which travel through the bloodstream to regulate various bodily functions like growth, metabolism, reproduction, and mood. It acts as a communication system between the different organs and tissues by sending hormonal signals. Let's meet some of the key players.

Scan for more information about the endocrine system.

All videos are provided courtesy of Alilia Medical Media. Copying and/ or downloading of any of the videos or animations to any social media platforms such as YouTube, Facebook, or TikTok is strictly prohibited.

©Alila Medical Media. All medical materials are for information purposes *only* and are *not* intended to be medical advice.

The **hypothalamus gland** is a small but critically important region located at the base of the brain, just above the pituitary gland. Despite its small size, the hypothalamus plays a central role in the regulation of the endocrine system, integrating signals from the nervous system and orchestrating the body's hormonal responses to maintain homeostasis. Think of it as the control center sending orders downstream to the master gland, the pituitary.

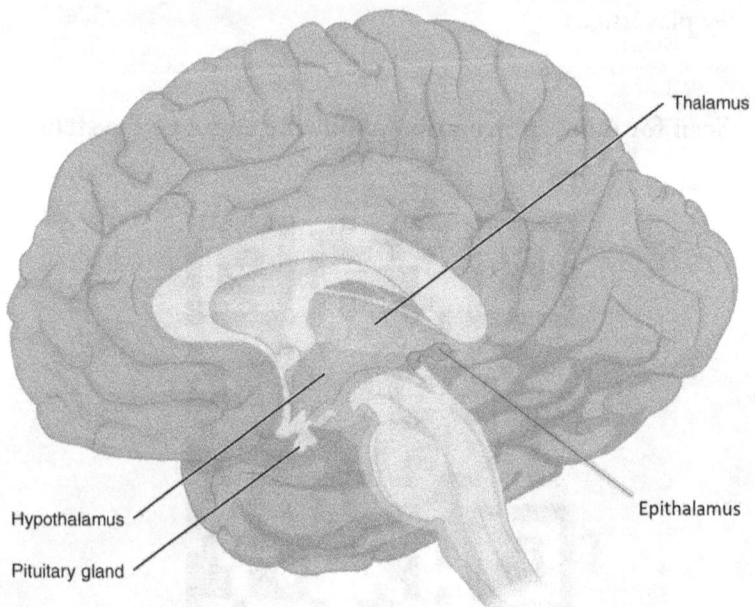

This Photo by Unknown Author is licensed under CC BY

- **Regulation of Hormone Release**
    » The hypothalamus controls the release of hormones from the pituitary gland, which in turn regulates many other endocrine glands in the body. It secretes hormones, which travel to the anterior pituitary gland to either stimulate or inhibit the release of hormones such as growth hormone (GH), thyroid-stimulating hormone (TSH), and adrenocorticotropic hormone (ACTH)

- **Homeostasis**
  - » The hypothalamus is critical for maintaining the body's internal balance, or homeostasis. It regulates key physiological processes such as body temperature, hunger, thirst, sleep, and circadian rhythms. By monitoring the internal environment of the body, the hypothalamus can trigger responses that help to correct any imbalances.
- **Stress Response**
  - » The hypothalamus plays a central role in the body's response to stress. It activates the hypothalamic-pituitary-adrenal (HPA) axis by releasing corticotropin-releasing hormone (CRH), which prompts the pituitary gland to secrete ACTH. ACTH then stimulates the adrenal glands to produce cortisol, a hormone that helps the body respond to stress.
- **Control of Reproductive Functions**
  - » The hypothalamus regulates reproductive functions through its control of the release of gonadotropin-releasing hormone (GnRH). GnRH stimulates the pituitary gland to release luteinizing hormone (LH) and follicle-stimulating hormone (FSH), which are essential for the regulation of the reproductive organs.

The **pituitary gland**, often called the "master conductor," is a pea-sized gland that is tucked away at the base of your brain, behind the bridge of the nose and directly below your hypothalamus. There are two main parts, or lobes: the anterior front lobe and the posterior back lobe. It orchestrates the activity of other glands by releasing hormones that regulate growth, metabolism, and reproductive functions, among other processes.

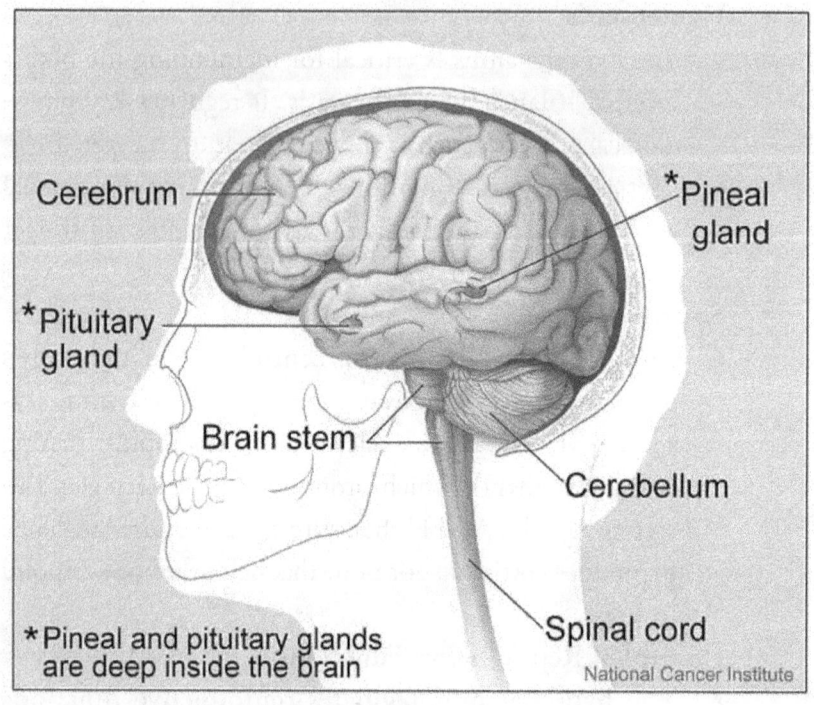

CC BY 4.0

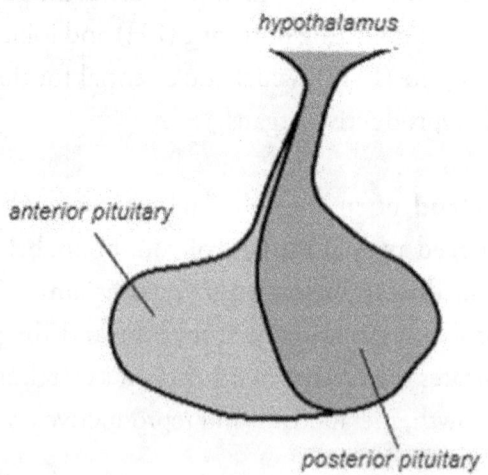

This Photo by Unknown Author is licensed under CC BY SA

The anterior pituitary makes and releases the following hormones:
- **Adrenocorticotrophic hormone (ACTH)**, which stimulates the adrenal glands to produce cortisol (the "stress hormone") which has many functions such as regulating metabolism, blood pressure, and blood sugar. It also plays a role in managing the immune system and the response to inflammation.
- **Thyroid-stimulating hormone (TSH)**, which stimulates the thyroid to produce thyroid hormones T4 and T3 which manage metabolism and energy levels. The pituitary gland produces TSH in response to the body's need for thyroid hormones. So when thyroid hormone levels fall too low, the pituitary gland releases more TSH to stimulate the thyroid gland.
- **Prolactin**, which stimulates breast milk production after childbirth, during breast development, and as part of other functions including metabolism and mood. It can also affect fertility and libido (sex drive) in adults. It is mainly controlled by a neurotransmitter called dopamine.
- **Growth hormone**, which stimulates growth of bones in children and maintains healthy bones and muscles in adults. It also impacts cell regeneration, carbohydrate metabolism, fat distribution, and how your body turns food into energy.
- **Follicle-stimulating hormone (FSH)**, which stimulates sperm production in men and estrogen production in women. It also assists in egg production in the ovaries. During puberty, it signals the ovaries and testes to begin producing hormones, leading to the development of sexual characteristics.
- **Luteinizing hormone (LH)**, which plays an important role in regulating the reproductive systems in both men and women. In men, it stimulates the testes to make testosterone, which is crucial for sperm production. In women, it triggers ovulation and promotes the production of progesterone.

The posterior pituitary makes and releases the hormones listed below.
- **Antidiuretic hormone (ADH)**, which regulates and balances water and sodium levels in the body. It works by increasing water reabsorption in the kidneys, helping the body retain water and maintain proper blood pressure.
- **Oxytocin** is stored and released during childbirth to assist in contracting the uterus during labor in women. In men, it helps move sperm. It is sometimes called the "love hormone" or "cuddle hormone" due to its role in social bonding and feelings of trust and affection.

Scan to learn more about the hypothalamus and pituitary glands.

All videos are provided courtesy of Alilia Medical Media. Copying and/or downloading of any of the videos or animations to any social media platforms such as YouTube, Facebook, or TikTok is strictly prohibited.

©Alila Medical Media. All medical materials are for information purposes *only* and are *not* intended to be medical advice.

The **pineal gland** is a small endocrine gland located deep within the brain. It plays a crucial role in regulating various physiological functions.

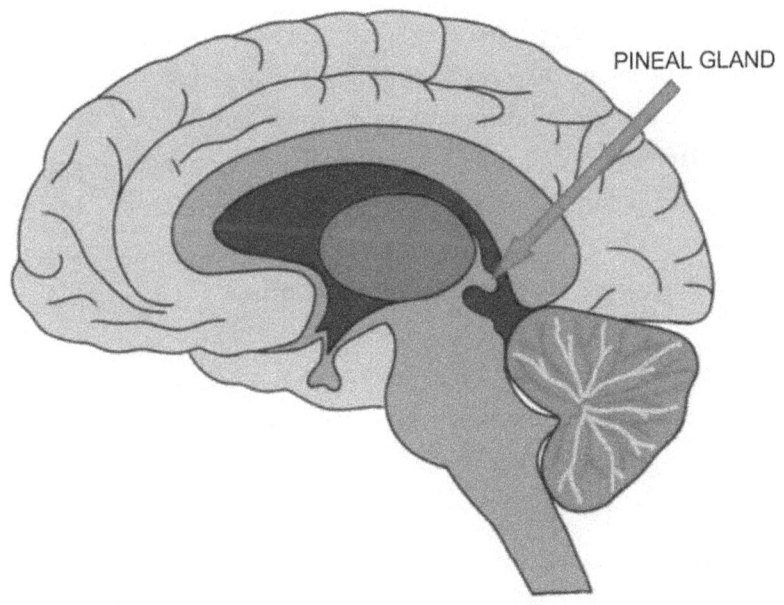

This Photo by Unknown Author is licensed under CC BY

Below is a summary of its primary functions.
- **Melatonin production:** The pineal gland's primary function is the production of melatonin, a hormone that regulates sleep-wake cycles. Melatonin secretion increases in response to darkness, helping to promote sleep, and decreases in the presence of light, aiding wakefulness.
- **Circadian rhythms:** By producing melatonin, the pineal gland helps synchronize the body's internal clock, or circadian rhythms, which govern sleep patterns, feeding behaviors, and other daily physiological cycles.

- **Reproductive function:** The pineal gland has been implicated in the regulation of reproductive hormones. Melatonin influences the timing of puberty and seasonal reproductive cycles in some animals.
- **Antioxidant properties:** Melatonin also acts as an antioxidant, protecting cells from damage by free radicals, thus contributing to the overall health and longevity of cells.
- **Immune system modulation:** There is evidence suggesting that the pineal gland, through its melatonin production, can modulate immune responses, potentially enhancing the body's defense mechanisms against pathogens.

The pineal gland is a small but mighty component of the endocrine system, essential for maintaining the balance of various bodily functions, particularly those related to sleep and circadian rhythms.

The **thyroid gland** is a butterfly-shaped gland located in your neck, below the Adam's apple. The thyroid sets the tempo for your metabolism, energy production, and even body temperature. It secretes two thyroid hormones—**thyroxine (T4) and triiodothyronine (T3)**—which influence metabolic rate, growth, and development. This, in turn, plays a role in controlling heart rate, muscle function, digestion, brain development, and bone maintenance. Its proper functioning depends on a good supply of iodine from the diet. It also secretes a peptide hormone called **calcitonin** which plays a role in calcium balance.

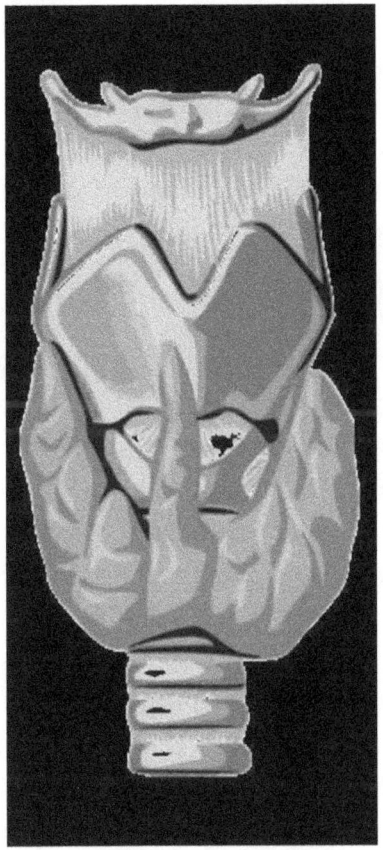

CC BY 4.0

- **Hormone Production**
    - » The primary function of the thyroid gland is to produce thyroid hormones, namely thyroxine (T4) and triiodothyronine (T3). These hormones are derived from iodine, which the thyroid gland absorbs from the bloodstream. T4 and T3 are released into the bloodstream where they regulate the metabolism of almost every cell in the body, influencing energy production, heat generation, and oxygen consumption.

- **Regulation of Metabolism**
  » Thyroid hormones play a pivotal role in regulating the body's metabolism. They control the rate at which the body converts food into energy and how efficiently cells use this energy. Higher levels of thyroid hormones increase the metabolic rate, while lower levels decrease it. This regulation affects body weight, heart rate, and overall energy levels.
- **Growth and Development**
  » The thyroid gland is essential for normal growth and development, especially in infants and children. Thyroid hormones are critical for brain development during the fetal stage and in early childhood. A deficiency in thyroid hormones during these stages can lead to intellectual disabilities and growth retardation.
- **Feedback Mechanism**
  » The thyroid gland is regulated by the hypothalamus and pituitary gland through a feedback loop. The hypothalamus secretes thyrotropin-releasing hormone (TRH), which stimulates the pituitary gland to release thyroid-stimulating hormone (TSH). TSH then prompts the thyroid gland to produce and release T3 and T4. When thyroid hormone levels are sufficient, they signal the hypothalamus and pituitary to reduce TRH and TSH production, thus maintaining hormonal balance.

Scan to learn more about the thyroid gland.

All videos are provided courtesy of Alilia Medical Media. Copying and/or downloading of any of the videos or animations to any social media platforms such as YouTube, Facebook, or TikTok is strictly prohibited.

©Alila Medical Media. All medical materials are for information purposes *only* and are *not* intended to be medical advice.

The **adrenal glands** are triangular-shaped glands located atop each of your kidneys. They keep the body functioning during stressful times by producing hormones that regulate stress responses, blood pressure, and fluid balance.

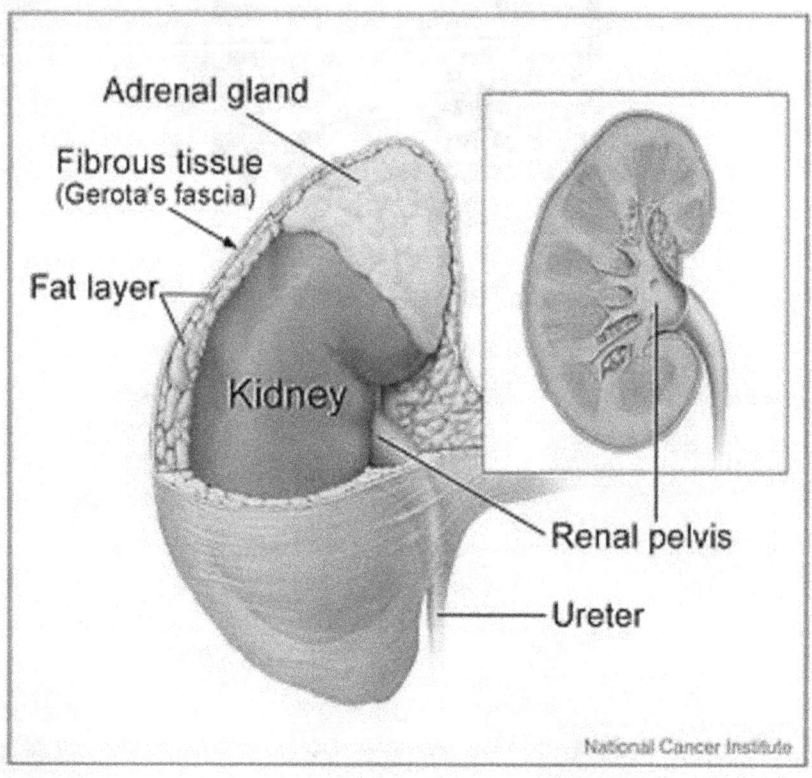

CC BY 4.0

The adrenal glands produce the following hormones.
- **Aldosterone**, which helps regulate blood pressure and electrolyte balance (especially potassium levels).
- **Cortisol and cortisone**, which help regulate metabolism and immune system suppression. It helps the body's use of fats, proteins, and carbohydrates. It also controls your sleep-wake cycle in a circadian rhythm. The release of cortisol helps the

Understanding Hormones and the Endocrine System

body get more energy in times of stress, such as when you are sick or in a car accident.
- **Androgens** like **DHEA and DHEAS** that are converted to fully functional sex hormones in the gonads.
- **Catecholamines (epinephrine and norepinephrine)** or "adrenaline," which help to produce a rapid "fight or flight" response throughout the body during physically and emotionally stressful situations. They increase heart rate and heart contractions to increase blood flow to your muscles and brain to help you get out of those dangerous situations. They also assist in glucose metabolism. They contract your blood vessels to help maintain blood pressure, thus preventing you from losing consciousness.

Scan to learn more about the adrenal glands.

All videos are provided courtesy of Alilia Medical Media. Copying and/or downloading of any of the videos or animations to any social media platforms such as YouTube, Facebook, or TikTok is strictly prohibited.

©Alila Medical Media. All medical materials are for information purposes *only* and are *not* intended to be medical advice.

The **pancreas** is a large, versatile gland located in the upper back of the abdomen with dual roles in the endocrine system and the digestive system. The pancreas functions as an endocrine gland as it maintains the harmony of your blood sugar levels through the release of **insulin** and **glucagon**. It also functions as an exocrine gland by producing enzymes to help with digestion.

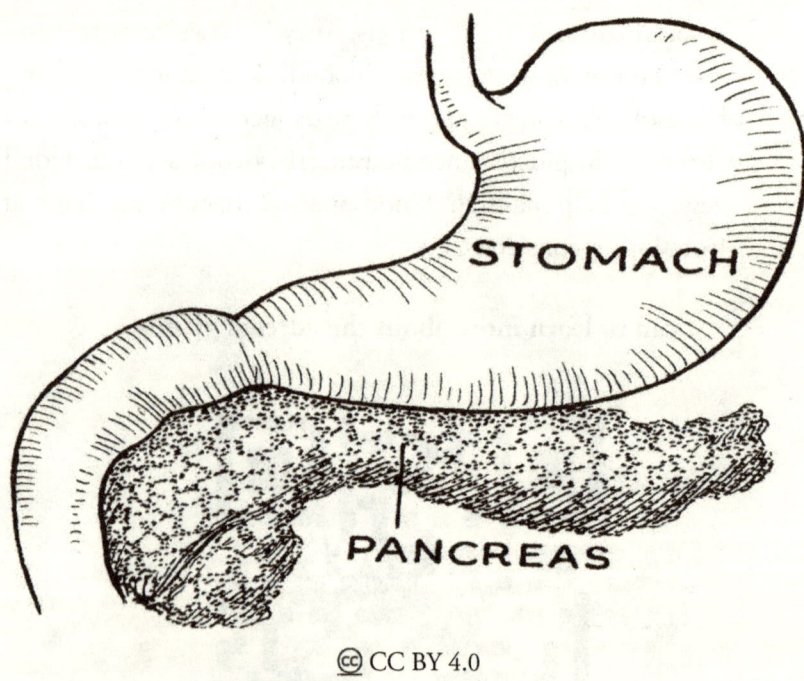

CC BY 4.0

- **Hormone Production**
    - » The pancreas contains clusters of cells known as the islets of Langerhans, which are responsible for its endocrine functions. The islets contain several types of cells, each producing specific hormones.
        - **Beta cells** produce insulin, a hormone essential for lowering blood glucose levels by promoting the uptake of glucose into cells.

- **Alpha cells** produce glucagon, a hormone that raises blood glucose levels by stimulating the liver to release stored glucose.
- **Delta cells** produce somatostatin, which regulates and inhibits the secretion of both insulin and glucagon.
- **PP cells** produce pancreatic polypeptides, which play a role in regulating the exocrine function of the pancreas and influences appetite.

- **Regulation of Blood Sugar Levels**
    » The primary role of pancreatic hormones is to maintain glucose homeostasis. After you eat, your pancreas secretes insulin in response to increased blood glucose levels. Insulin facilitates the uptake of glucose into cells, where it can be used for energy or stored as glycogen in the liver and muscles. Conversely, when blood glucose levels drop, such as during fasting, glucagon is secreted to stimulate the release of glucose from glycogen stores, ensuring a steady supply of energy.
- **Role in Metabolism**
    » Beyond glucose regulation, insulin also plays a role in fat and protein metabolism. It promotes the storage of fats in adipose tissue and inhibits the breakdown of fat stores. It also aids in protein synthesis by facilitating the uptake of amino acids into cells. Glucagon, on the other hand, encourages the breakdown of fats into fatty acids and the conversion of proteins into glucose through gluconeogenesis.

Pancreatic Disorders

- **Diabetes mellitus:** The most well-known disorder associated with the pancreas is diabetes mellitus, a condition characterized by impaired insulin production or action. Type 1 diabetes results from the autoimmune destruction of beta cells, leading to little or no insulin production. Type 2 diabetes is characterized by insulin resistance, where cells fail to respond adequately to insulin, leading to high blood sugar levels.

- **Pancreatitis:** Inflammation of the pancreas, known as pancreatitis, can interfere with both its endocrine and exocrine functions. Chronic pancreatitis can lead to diabetes if the insulin-producing cells are damaged.

Scan to learn more about the pancreas.

All videos are provided courtesy of Alilia Medical Media. Copying and/or downloading of any of the videos or animations to any social media platforms such as YouTube, Facebook, or TikTok is strictly prohibited.

©Alila Medical Media. All medical materials are for information purposes *only* and are *not* intended to be medical advice.

The **ovaries** are small, oval-shaped glands located on each side of the uterus. They produce and store eggs for reproduction and make the hormones **estrogen** and **progesterone** that control the menstrual cycle and pregnancy.

The **testes** (testicles) are responsible for making sperm for reproduction and producing a hormone called **testosterone** which helps with muscle development, deepening of the voice, and growing body hair.

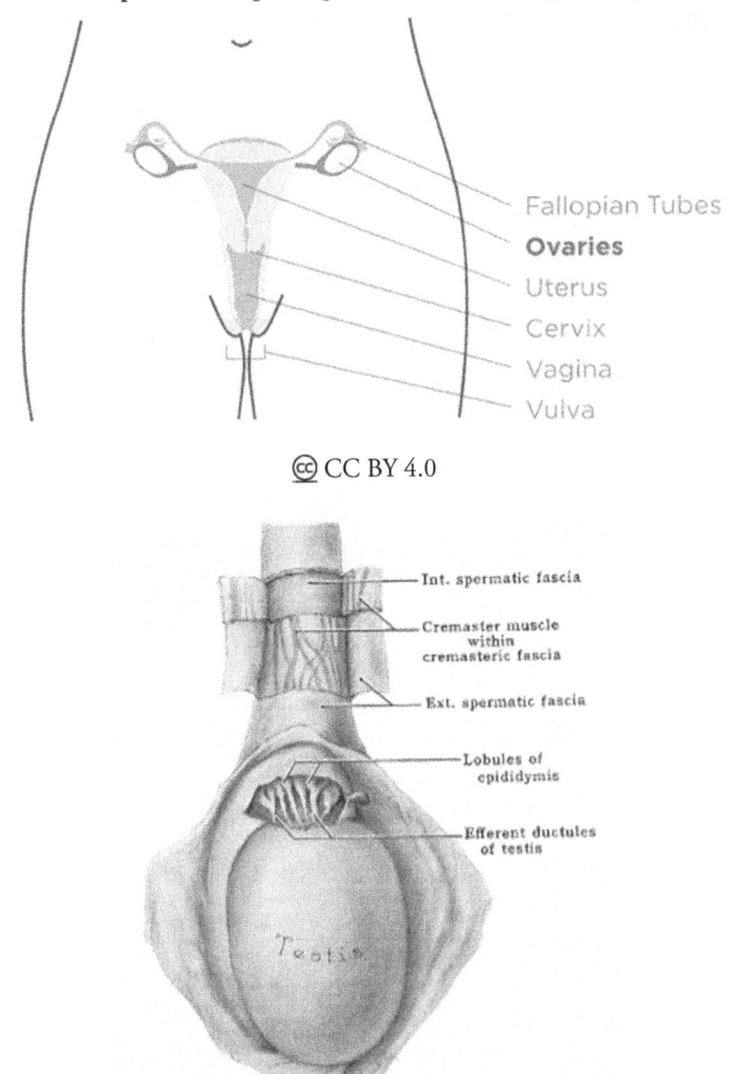

CC BY 4.0

CC BY 4.0

This may be a shock to most of you, but **adipose tissue (fat cells)** is part of the endocrine system. It is complex and functions as an integrated unit to store excess energy. It responds to different signals but also secretes factors with important endocrine functions. These factors include **leptin, adiponectin, plasminogen activator inhibitor-1, proteins of the renin-angiotensin system**, and **resistin**. Adipose tissue is also a major site for metabolism of sex steroids and glucocorticoids like cortisol.

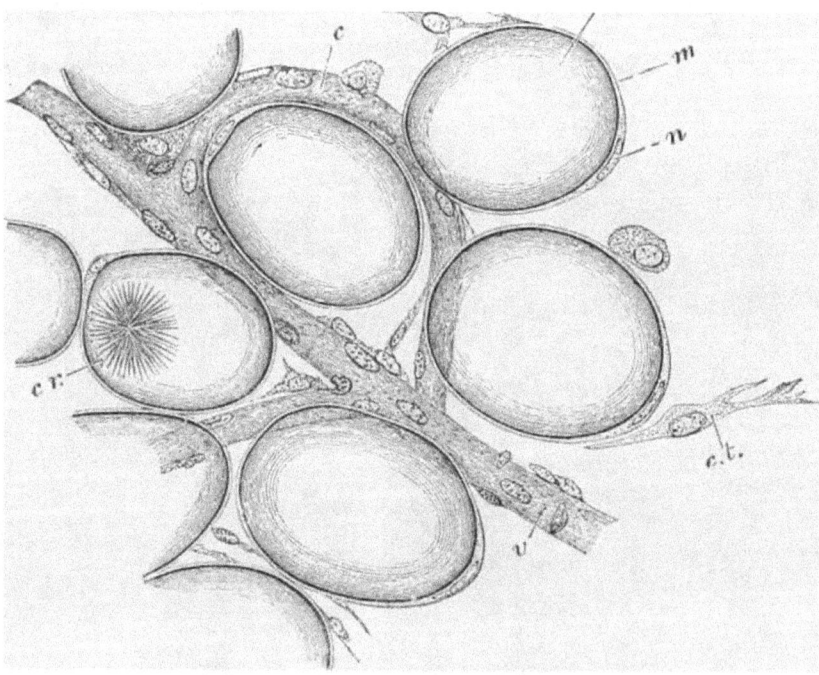

CC BY 4.0

The Art of Hormonal Balance: Feedback Loops

Maintaining the harmony of this hormonal symphony is a delicate art. Your body relies on feedback loops to keep hormone levels in check.

Most commonly, the system uses a negative feedback loop, which works like a thermostat.

Let's image that your house is too chilly. The smart thermostat (in this scenario, the hypothalamus) notices the temperature is too low. It sends a message through the app (pituitary gland) to turn on the heater (thyroid gland). The heater kicks on and warms the house (releasing T3 and T4 thyroid hormones). Once the temperature rises to the right level, the thermostat sees this and stops sending commands. The heater slows down, keeping your body cozy with the temperature just right. This is called a negative feedback loop—a built-in safety check to keep things from going too high or too low.

When hormone levels sway too high or too low, the body orchestrates a series of reactions to bring them back to equilibrium. Another example is when there is a rise in blood sugar, which will prompt the pancreas to release insulin, helping to lower sugar levels; conversely, if sugar levels dip, glucagon is released to elevate them. The negative feedback loop keeps things in check.

On the other hand, positive feedback loops work to escalate specific processes. In events like childbirth, the hormone oxytocin ramps up contractions until the baby is delivered. It's like getting a group text message that just won't stop. The body gets a text during childbirth: "Hey, we're in labor! Bring on the oxytocin!" The brain then sends group text: "I'm releasing the oxytocin to get those contractions going." Contractions signal the brain to release *more* oxytocin. This cycle continues over and over until the baby is delivered. Then you get the numerous "Yes!" responses in the group text until the event is over. Finally, the positive feedback loop is complete.

Here are two other examples of these feedback loops.

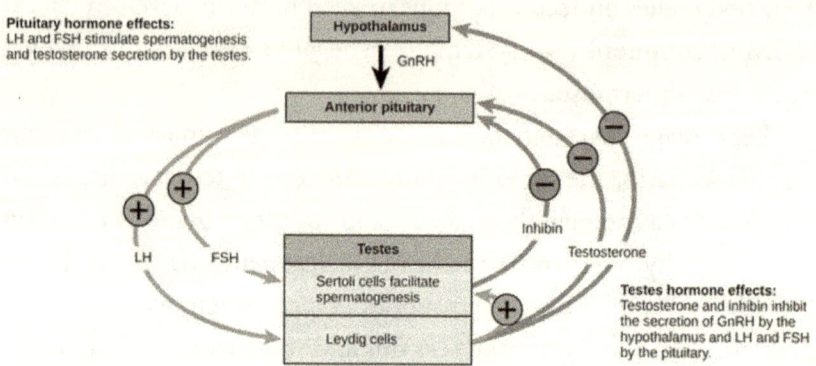

This Photo by Unknown Author is licensed under CC BY-SA

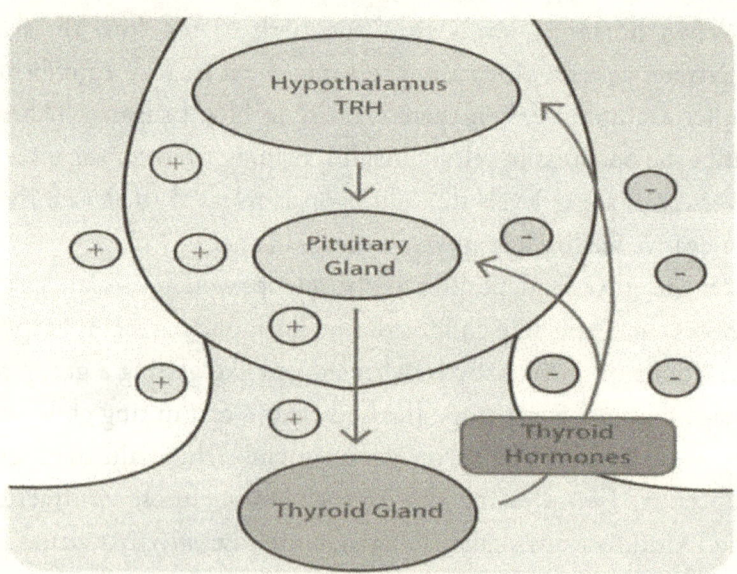

This Photo by Unknown Author is licensed under CC BY-SA

Conclusion

So I hope you now know your ABC's about hormones and how they work. You can see that the human body has so much more than just estrogen and testosterone. With this knowledge as our foundation, we can now delve into how EDCs affect our hormones. Understanding the fascinating world of hormones and the endocrine system helps us truly grasp the dangers of EDCs. In the upcoming chapters, we'll explore exactly how EDCs affect our health, and we'll learn practical strategies to minimize their impact and improve our well-being.

CHAPTER TWO:

What the Heck Are Endocrine-Disrupting Chemicals (EDCs)?

You are now stepping into the complex and sometimes unsettling landscape of endocrine-disrupting chemicals, or EDCs for short. So, what exactly are these mysterious substances, and why should you be concerned? Let me break it down for you and demystify EDCs and their impact on our well-being.

EDCs 101: More than Just a Chemical or Toxin

EDCs are the troublemakers of the chemical world. These substances, whether they are man-made or natural, affect your endocrine system by having a disposition to disrupt it, something we looked at in chapter one. The problem with these chemical culprits is that they are present almost everywhere—in industrial chemicals, pesticides, plastics, pharmaceuticals, and even some personal care products.

What makes EDCs so challenging is that they don't come with one set of problems. They are packed with many different ways of disrupting your hormones and causing chaos in your body. They can function as endocrine disrupters by acting as hormone mimics, by competing with hormone receptors, or by interfering with the secretion and actions of hormones. Thus, they can disrupt the endocrine system and lead to various health issues.

Think of your body as a high-security building, with hormones acting as authorized employees who carry out critical jobs to keep everything running smoothly at the company: temperature, mood, sleep, metabolism, fertility, and more.

Now imagine EDCs as imposters who have fake badges and are trying to sneak into this building. They don't just break in one way; they've got a whole list of choices for how to break into the building. So as the true hormones (estrogen, testosterone, thyroid hormones, and others) come in with their ID badges, security (your hormone receptors) scans each badge and lets them in. However, the EDC imposters soon enter. Scenario one is that they can impersonate the real hormones. "Hello, I'm estrogen!" These chemicals look similar enough to the real hormones that the body gets fooled. They sneak past security and trigger reactions the body didn't ask for. This leads to confusion while signaling fire when they shouldn't. Scenario two is that they block the real hormones. They park in the spaces meant for actual hormones. This prevents the real ones from getting to work. Important jobs go undone and systems begin to fail. Scenario three is that they disrupt hormone production. They distract or fool the security guards (the hormone receptors) and tamper with the factory. This leads to a change in how much hormone is made; either too much or too little. The body's delicate balance gets thrown off. Scenario four is that they interfere with the messaging system. As they come into the building, their fake badges get scanned and release a virus that infects the whole computer system. Much like hackers, they disrupt the communication lines between glands. The wrong instructions get sent, or none are sent at all. This causes confusion across the hormonal network, which in time can cause total shutdown. EDCs are master impersonators and hackers. They can slip into our hormone systems, disrupt security, hijack messages, and leave behind a trail of chaos.

This is illustrated in figure A below, where the EDC in pink is blocking the receptor in blue. It can also stop the binding of the normal hormone (in green) to the receptor. However, in figure B, the EDC can act like the natural hormone and bind directly to the receptor.

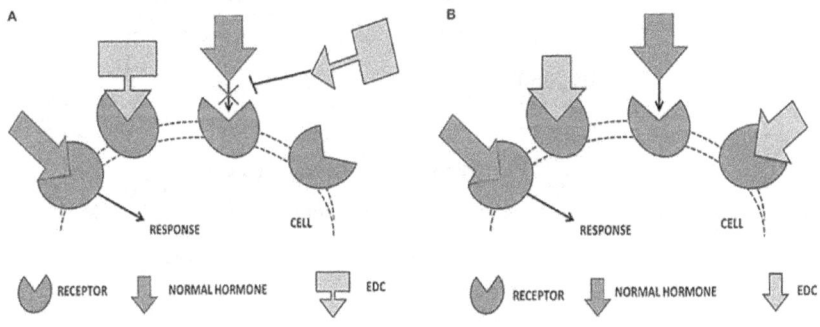

This Photo by Unknown Author is licensed under CC BY

EDCs and Your Health: A Pandora's Box

The health ramifications of EDC exposure are startling and wide-ranging. These chemicals have been implicated in a host of issues, including:
- Hormone-sensitive cancers like breast, prostate, and testicular cancers
- Reproductive problems and fertility issues
- Developmental abnormalities in children
- Thyroid dysfunctions
- Metabolic problems like obesity and diabetes
- Immune system glitches
- Neurological and behavioral disorders, including impacts on cognitive function

What makes EDCs particularly concerning is their ability to cause havoc even at minuscule levels—levels that are often deemed as safe by regulatory agencies. This is especially problematic for vulnerable populations (such as unborn babies, infants, and young children) whose rapid growth and development make them particularly sensitive to even the tiniest hormonal fluctuations.

Below is a summarized table of some of the more commonly recognized EDCs and their primary sites or modes of action based on available scientific literature.

EDC	Primary Site/Mode of Action
Bisphenol A (BPA)	Estrogen receptors, thyroid hormone signaling
Phthalates	Androgen (male sex hormone) signaling, reproductive system
Polychlorinated biphenyls (PCBs)	Thyroid hormone pathways, neurological development
Polybrominated diphenyl ethers (PBDEs)	Thyroid hormone disruption, neurodevelopment
Dioxins	AHR (aryl hydrocarbon receptor) pathway, immune system
Perfluorooctanoic acid (PFOA)	Liver, thyroid, immune system, developmental processes
Perfluorooctanesulfonic acid (PFOS)	Liver, thyroid, immune system, cholesterol metabolism
Atrazine	Hypothalamic-pituitary-gonadal axis, estrogen and testosterone levels
Lead	Neurodevelopment, calcium signaling
Arsenic	Hormone signaling pathways, glucose metabolism
Mercury	Neurological and hormonal pathways, developmental processes
Dichloro-diphenyl-trichloroethane (DDT)	Estrogen receptor, reproductive and neurological systems

EDC	Primary Site/Mode of Action
Glyphosate	Aromatase enzyme, androgen and estrogen biosynthesis
Organophosphate pesticides	Neurotransmitter systems, hormonal disruptions
Parabens	Estrogen receptors, skin, breast tissue
Triclosan	Thyroid hormone signaling, bacterial resistance mechanisms
Tributyltin (TBT)	Retinoid X receptor and peroxisome proliferator-activated receptors, obesity and metabolism issues
Hexachlorobenzene (HCB)	Thyroid hormone pathways, immune system disruptions
Bisphenol S (BPS)	Estrogen receptors, similar endocrine-disrupting properties as BPA

Explanation of Table

- **Bisphenol A (BPA)** and **phthalates** are used in plastics and can mimic or block hormones.
- **PCBs** and **PBDEs** are used as industrial lubricants and flame retardants, respectively, and interfere with thyroid hormones and neurodevelopment.
- **Dioxins**, unintentional by-products of combustion processes, activate specific receptors leading to diverse toxicological effects.
- **Perfluorooctanoic acid (PFOA)** and **perfluorooctanesulfonic acid (PFOS)** are part of the PFAS family, widely used in nonstick coatings and water-repellent materials. They are linked to multiple health issues, including hormonal imbalances and liver toxicity.

- **Perfluoroalkyl substances (PFAS)** are used in nonstick coatings and affect multiple systems, including liver and immune function.
- **Atrazine**, an herbicide, disrupts reproductive hormones.
- Heavy metals like **lead**, **arsenic**, and **mercury** interfere with brain development and hormone pathways.
- **DDT**, a banned pesticide, still persists in the environment and affects estrogenic pathways.
- **Glyphosate**, a widely used herbicide, impacts hormonal synthesis.
- **Organophosphate pesticides** affect neurotransmitter functions and hormonal balance.
- **Parabens** and **triclosan** are used in cosmetics and personal care products and can mimic estrogen or disrupt thyroid function.
- **Tributyltin (TBT)** is used as an antifouling agent in paints for ships and as a wood preservative. It's particularly notorious for promoting adipogenesis, leading to obesity in exposed organisms, a phenomenon known as the "obesogen" effect.
- **Hexachlorobenzene (HCB)**, once used as a pesticide and a by-product of industrial processes, is known to cause thyroid and immune system problems.
- **Bisphenol S (BPS)** is often used as a substitute for BPA in "BPA-free" products; however, emerging research suggests that BPS also disrupts endocrine functions in similar ways to BPA, affecting estrogen pathways and potentially leading to reproductive and developmental issues.

Where Are These EDCs Hiding?

You would be surprised at the many avenues through which EDCs can sneak into your life.

Environmental pollution: Industrial and agricultural activities often release EDCs into the air, soil, and water, creating a contaminated backdrop to our lives.

Food and drink: Pesticides on produce; hormones in meat, vegetable oil, soy products, and store-canned foods; and chemicals in packaging can introduce EDCs right into your diet.

Everyday products: Think your home is safe? EDCs often lurk in plastics, personal care products like lotions and soaps, cleaning agents, fragranced candles, plastic storage containers, Teflon pots and pans, conventional pads and tampons, and even items treated with flame retardants.

Medications: Some pharmaceuticals and synthetic multivitamins, especially hormonal treatments, can act as EDCs either when they find their way into the environment or when misused.

On the job: Certain professions in manufacturing, agriculture, health care, and lab work may expose workers to higher EDC levels.

Conclusion

So, to recap, EDCs are the uninvited guests in our bodies. They interfere with many aspects of hormone function and action. They can either mimic—and thus replace—naturally occurring hormones, interfere with hormone transport to target organs, bind to hormone receptors to prevent hormone action, or block hormone secretion and production. As a result, they can disrupt hormonal balance, affecting everything from developmental milestones to the risk of chronic diseases. They have been linked to numerous hormonal disorders that lead to weight gain, depression, anxiety, thyroid disease, reproductive issues, insulin resistance, PCOS, obesity, infertility, brain fog, diabetes, fibroids, allergies, and cancer.

The impacts of EDCs can have short-term as well as long-term implications. For example, exposure during critical periods, like fetal development, can lead to lifelong repercussions, affecting fertility, mental development, and metabolic health. EDCs have also been linked to conditions such as obesity, thyroid issues, cancers of the breast and prostate, and weakened immune systems. It is essential to know what EDCs are and where they come from to avoid the risks to our endocrine health.

In the following chapters, we will look more closely at the effects of these chemicals on our health, discuss the latest findings, and, most importantly, help you to reduce your exposure to these substances and look after your health. Stay tuned!

CHAPTER THREE:

Comprehending the Impact of EDCs and Their Link to Various Illnesses and Health Conditions

Endocrine-disrupting chemicals (EDCs) are the chemicals that are as friendly as wolves in sheep's clothing. They can enter your body and play havoc with your endocrine system. These chemicals can be found in plastics, pesticides, personal care products, and pharmaceuticals, among other products. Although they may appear harmless, EDCs are known to act like estrogen, androgen, or thyroid stimulators or blockers, thus disturbing your normal hormonal functions and leading to several health issues. As we discussed in the first two chapters, hormones are the body's messengers that regulate almost all of the functions: metabolic, growth, reproduction, and immunity. If you are exposed to EDCs, they will interfere with these signals and can affect almost every part of your health. The impact can be widespread; they can affect how your organs function, the state of your tissues, and even how you feel emotionally.

The impacts from EDCs reach far beyond their effects on humans. The consequences on wildlife and the environment are vastly underappreciated. EDCs have been shown to interfere with reproductive processes in wildlife, leading to altered hormone levels and reduced fertility. The cumulative effects lead to declines in population sizes and shifts in species diversity. This creates a domino effect that disrupts the ecosystem and potentially affects the nutrients in the food supply. Some EDCs can accumulate in the tissues of seafood, especially in larger fish. In addition, pharmaceuticals (like antibiotics and hormones) have been found in the environment through wastewater treatment plants. Since drinking tap water is a potential source of human exposure to EDCs, numerous studies worldwide have detected and confirmed the prevalence of these chemicals.

Furthermore, the financial impact is estimated to have a serious threat to public health and a burden on US health-care costs. NYU Langone Health says, "Exposure to endocrine-disrupting chemicals (EDCs) has major economic consequences because of the diseases they cause. The healthcare costs and lost earnings caused by EDC exposure have been calculated to cost the European Union about €157 billion every year (about $209 billion), which is approximately 1.23% of the EU's gross domestic product." The economic burden is higher in the United States, however. A study in *The Lancet Diabetes & Endocrinology* estimated that the annual health-care costs and lost earnings of daily low-level exposure to EDCs is $340 billion and greater than 2.3 percent of the US gross domestic product. Also, a study conducted on the effects of EDCs present in plastics and their impact on public health was published in the *Journal of the Endocrine Society*. These figures highlight the overall economic burden of the health complications that are associated with EDC exposure, and therefore demonstrate the importance of regulatory measures and public health interventions to prevent exposure and avoid the associated costs. One of the most significant impacts of EDCs is on reproductive health. They don't discriminate—both males and females are affected. Phthalates and bisphenol-A (BPA) are chemicals that have been linked to low sperm count and motility in men. These chemicals can lead to irregular menstruation and infertility and can affect ovulation in women. Further, if a pregnant woman is exposed to EDCs, these chemicals can interfere with the reproductive development of the fetus and cause long-term health complications. The effects of EDC exposure are not only limited to reproductive health. Neurodevelopmental disorders like ADHD, cognitive delays, and behavioral problems can also be triggered in children if they are exposed to these chemicals at the critical stages of their development. However, most of these effects persist through adulthood and affect brain function and quality of life. The use of EDCs is also being watched closely due to their potential to cause hormone-related cancers. Some of these chemicals are estrogenic and can increase the risk of growth of breast and ovarian cancers. Thus, EDCs act via binding to hormone receptors and may accelerate growth of cancer cells of concern. Metabolically, EDCs are known to disrupt blood sugar and fat metabolism and increase the risk of obesity and type 2 diabetes. As such, the role that EDCs play in these conditions cannot be ruled out as metabolic disorders are on the rise globally. Your immune system, the body's defense against disease, is not immune to the effects of EDCs. These chemicals can suppress your immune system and make you more prone to diseases, autoimmune diseases, and allergies. At one time, EDCs were thought to be harmless. However, scientists have now proven that these chemicals are dangerous and should be avoided as much as possible. In the next chapter, we will dig deeper to learn more about the various illnesses caused by EDCs.

CHAPTER FOUR:

How EDCs Are Making Us Sick: The Effects of EDCs on Health

After getting a grasp of the basics about EDCs and the various health risks linked to them, let's delve into their impact in developing diseases. As an endocrinologist, my expertise focuses on how these EDCs cause hormonal disruption. However, I wanted to highlight the broader health consequences. In this chapter, we'll explore how EDCs contribute to both acute and chronic medical issues, and we'll unveil their links to long-lasting ailments. The goal is to offer an examination of how EDCs exhibit their impact on human health, even at a molecular level.

Acute Exposure: The Immediate Dangers

While much attention is focused on the chronic impact of EDCs, we shouldn't overlook the immediate risks posed by acute exposure. These can include the following issues.

Allergic Reactions
Skin irritations and allergic reactions: Certain chemicals, like parabens and phthalates, present in beauty and personal grooming items have been known to trigger skin problems for some people. These issues can vary from annoyances like redness and itching to serious allergic reactions such as hives or eczema. The skin acts like a shield, defending the body against harmful substances. However, it can show a heightened reaction to chemical exposures, especially in individuals with sensitive skin or preexisting allergies.

Respiratory Issues
Exacerbation of asthma and respiratory conditions: Environmental chemicals, such as benzene and formaldehyde, found in air pollution can worsen respiratory problems. People with asthma or COPD may have flare-ups with wheezing, difficulty breathing, and cough. Being suddenly exposed to amounts of these pollutants can cause breathing difficulties in sensitive groups, like kids and seniors.

Digestive Upset
Gastrointestinal issues: EDCs such as pesticides, bisphenol A (BPA), and heavy metals in contaminated food or water can trigger gastrointestinal issues like queasiness and stomach cramps, in addition to other symptoms such as vomiting and diarrhea. These reactions stem from the body's response to ingested poisons that can upset the stomach lining and interfere with digestion processes. In some situations, exposure to toxins could lead to dehydration that may necessitate attention.

Chronic Exposure: The Silent Scourge
Extended exposure to EDCs raises concerns for the following reasons.

Hormonal imbalance: As time passes, the impacts of EDCs build up, causing lasting irregularities in hormone levels which may result in ailments such as hypothyroidism and conditions like polycystic ovarian syndrome (PCOS) and insulin resistance (which will be further explored in chapters five and six).

Inflammation: When we hear about inflammation, we often automatically think of arthritis or the skin's reaction to an insect bite. However, it is not well known that inflammation is the root of so many problems, even weight gain. EDCs have been shown to trigger chronic inflammation, resulting in various diseases such as heart conditions and specific types of cancer.

As seen in the diagram below, EDCs can promote the development of larger fat cells which, in turn, store toxins and inhibit our metabolism. They disrupt our immune cells, increasing our susceptibility to autoimmune disorders. After chronic exposure, an imbalance of free radicals can increase oxidative stress, thus leading to chronic disease such as heart disease, premature aging, Alzheimer's disease, cancer, and diabetes. Lastly, genetic mutations can occur, making us prone to neurological diseases like Alzheimer's disease, developmental disorders, and cancer.

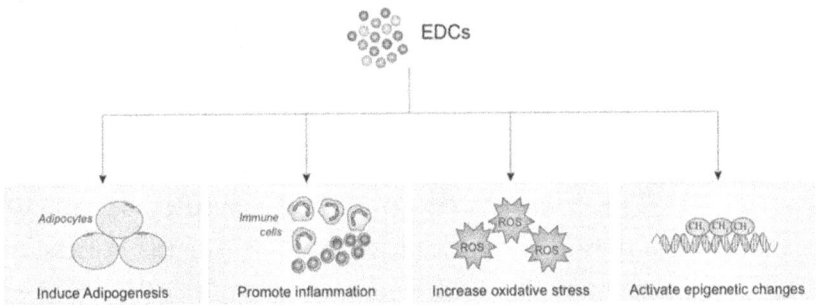

This Photo by Unknown Author is licensed under CC BY

- **EDCs and Inflammatory Markers: Prostaglandins, COX-1, COX-2, and CRP**
  » Inflammation plays a role in our system's normal protective and healing responses. However, persistent inflammation has been associated with a variety of health conditions. Prostaglandins and the enzymes cyclooxygenase (COX-1 and COX-2) and C-reactive protein (CRP) are important factors in the process of inflammation. Endocrine-disrupting chemicals can have a significant impact on these markers of inflammation, resulting in a range of health challenges.
- **Effects of EDCs on Inflammatory Markers**

1. **Prostaglandins:** Prostaglandins are molecules that play a role in causing inflammation and pain, as well as regulating body temperature by inducing fever symptoms. The presence of endocrine-disrupting chemicals (EDCs) like BPA and phthalates can influence the enzymes for prostaglandin synthesis, leading to an increase in prostaglandin production. Higher levels of prostaglandins can contribute to the development of inflammation. They are associated with health conditions such as arthritis and heart disease (Vélez et al. 2016). This why we use antiprostaglandins like aspirin and nonsteroidal anti-inflammatory drugs like Advil and Motrin to help treat arthritis.

2. **Cyclooxygenase (COX-1 and COX-2) enzymes:** COX-1 and COX-2 are the enzymes responsible for converting arachidonic acid to prostaglandins. EDCs can upregulate the expression and activity of these enzymes. For example, BPA increases COX-2 expression, leading to heightened prostaglandin synthesis and inflammation. Continual stimulation of COX-2 has been linked to conditions like cancer and inflammatory bowel disease like Crohn's disease. (Kassotis et al. 2015).

3. **C-reactive protein (CRP):** CRP is a key systemic inflammation marker produced by the liver. It has been shown that higher levels of BPA in the urine correlate with increased CRP levels, indicating chronic inflammation. Elevated CRP levels are associated with an increased risk of diseases such as atherosclerosis and hypertension. Atherosclerosis is the buildup of fats, cholesterol, and other substances in and on the artery walls. Collectively, this buildup is called plaque (Sabanayagam et al. 2013).

Understanding the Link Between Elevated Inflammatory Markers and the Development of Illnesses

1. **Cardiovascular diseases:** Cardiovascular diseases are influenced by inflammation as shown by levels of CRP and prostaglandins that play a role in the progression of atherosclerosis—a condition characterized by the accumulation of plaques in arteries that can result in heart attacks and strokes. Enhanced COX-2 expression, alongside inflammation, can worsen these plaques and increase the risk of rupture, leading to heart attacks (Libby et al. 2002).
2. **Cancer:** Evidence suggests that long-term exposure to chemicals could contribute to the growth and spread of cancer. Increasing COX-2 levels in the body can promote tumor development and spread to parts of the body. Long-term inflammation can also contribute to cancer by harming DNA to encourage blood vessel formation and weakening the system. Elevated levels of prostaglandins may stimulate the growth of cancer cells while preventing their natural cell death process, ultimately advancing the progression of cancer (Wang and DuBois 2010).

3. **Autoimmune diseases:** Autoimmune disorders can be worsened by EDCs as they can raise indicators such as prostaglandins and COX-2 expression, provoking inflammation and damage. Conditions like rheumatoid arthritis and lupus syndrome have been linked with high CRP levels and associated with disease exacerbations and heightened severity in autoimmune disorders (Firestein 2003).
4. **Metabolic disorders:** Chronic inflammation caused by levels of CRP and prostaglandins is associated with insulin resistance and type 2 diabetes. Molecules known as cytokines may interfere with insulin-signaling pathways, resulting in higher blood sugar levels and metabolic irregularities. This resistance to insulin triggered by inflammation plays a role in the emergence of metabolic syndrome (HotamisligiI et al. 2006).

Cellular changes: Some EDCs can cause DNA mutations or epigenetic changes that may increase the risk of cancers and other long-term diseases.

- **The Influence of Endocrine-Disrupting Chemicals on Stem Cells**
  - » Stem cells are cells that have not yet specialized and can transform into different types of cells. In the body, they aid in growth and development, and they play a crucial role in repairing and regenerating tissues and organs. However, EDCs can disrupt the functions of these stem cells, resulting in health problems.

- **Effects of EDCs on Stem Cells**
  - » **Disruption of stem cell differentiation:** EDCs can impact how stem cells develop into specific cell types. For

example, bisphenol A (known as BPA) has the potential to disrupt the differentiation of stem cells which could possibly impact brain development and functioning (Palanza et al. 2008). You can image how this can affect infants and children.

» **Altered stem cell proliferation:** EDCs can influence the rate at which stem cells proliferate. Phthalates are known to affect how stem cells multiply and grow in types of stem cells which could affect the process of tissue regeneration and repair (Martínez-Iglesias et al. 2010). So if they slow the growth of stem cells, the body is hampered from repairing itself.

» **Epigenetic modifications:** Endocrine-disruptive substances have the potential to cause alterations in stem cells by modifying gene expression without altering the DNA sequence itself. This transformation can impact the lasting performance of stem cells and their capacity to differentiate correctly (Manikkam et al. 2012). This can either inadvertently activate normally silent genes or suppress normally active genes responsible for various functions.

» **Stem cell niche disruption:** The environment surrounding stem cells also play a role in their performance and effectiveness. This ecosystem can be negatively impacted by EDCs, which may result in compromised stem cell functionality and contribute to conditions like cancer and metabolic disorders (Soto and Sonnenschein 2010).

- **Health Implications**
1. **Cancer:** EDCs have the potential to trigger the change of stem cells into cancer stem cells which, in turn, play a role in

starting and advancing tumors, especially in hormone-related cancers like breast and prostate cancer.
2. **Neurodevelopmental disorders:** Neurodevelopmental disorders can arise when EDCs interfere with the process of stem cell differentiation, and can result in conditions like autism and ADHD, especially if exposure happens during stages of brain development.
3. **Metabolic disorders:** Endocrine-disrupting chemicals (EDCs) have the potential to affect how mesenchymal stem cells develop into cells, which can play a role in causing obesity and other metabolic disorders by changing how fat is distributed and affecting metabolic balance.
4. **Reproductive health:** Reproductive health may be impacted by exposure to EDCs as they can influence germ line stem cells for producing sperm and eggs. This, in turn, potentially leads to issues like decreased fertility and increased risks of miscarriages and birth defects.

- **EDCs and Senescent Cells: Impact on Health**
  - » Senescent cells are cells that have stopped dividing yet continue to function within the body's processes. It is a response to various stressors, including DNA damage and oxidative stress. The definition of oxidative stress is when there are too many free radicals and not enough antioxidants to neutralize them, leading to damage to cellular components. This, in turn, damages the DNA, proteins, and other cellular structures. Senescent cells are involved in the aging process and the onset of age-related ailments such as cancer, heart disease, and dementia. While they may offer advantages like facilitating wound recovery, having an excess of these cells usually leads to

outcomes by promoting inflammation and impairments with tissue function. It should be noted that a diet high in sugar and carbohydrates, as well as overeating, can lead to an increased senescence burden. On the other hand, a restrictive diet or intermittent fasting may reduce the number of senescent cells. You will learn more about the benefits of intermittent fasting in chapter twelve.

- **The Impact of Endocrine-Disrupting Chemicals on Aging Cells**
1. **Induction of cellular senescence:** Cellular senescence can be prompted by EDCs, resulting in premature aging and impaired function in cells (Lee et al. 2019). Substances such as BPA and phthalates can induce DNA harm, oxidative stress, and mitochondrial dysfunction that activates pathways linked to senescence. Mitochondria are the powerhouses where nutrients are converted into energy. So as our cells age, so, too, do our bodies slowly deteriorate.
2. **Inflammatory secretions:** Senescent cells release substances (such as inflammatory cytokines and growth factors known as the senescence associated secretory phenotype, or SASP) that promote inflammation. Exposure to EDCs can worsen this reaction, leading to inflammation and harm to tissues (Tabas and Glass 2013).
3. **Impaired tissue regeneration:** Impaired tissue regeneration can occur due to the buildup of senescent cells which can hinder the ability of stem cells and progenitor cells to efficiently regenerate tissues (Van Deursen 2014). Our bodies become less efficient or equipped to defend or repair against offending agents.

4. **Promotion of tumorigenesis:** Although senescent cells can prevent tumor growth by stopping cell division, the inflammatory setting they produce may also adversely encourage tumorigenesis development. This is the process by which normal cells transform into cancerous ones with malignant properties like uncontrolled growth and spread. Therefore, EDCs might play a function in cancer progression by triggering senescence and nurturing an environment for tumor growth (Childs et al. 2015).

- **The Role of Environmental Disruptors and Telomeres in Stem Cells, and Their Effects on Overall Health**
  » Telomeres are protective caps at the ends of chromosomes, guarding them from damage and ensuring proper cell division. They are like the plastic tips on the ends of shoelaces, ensuring that the DNA strands don't fray or become damaged during cell division. Over time, telomeres shorten, leading to cellular aging and dysfunction. This is a natural process but may be hastened by external factors. Telomere length is crucial for maintaining stem cell function and overall cellular health.

- **Effects of EDCs on Telomeres in Stem Cells**
1. **Telomere shortening:** EDCs can speed up the shortening of telomeres by causing stress and DNA damage in the body. Chemicals like BPA and phthalates have been found to raise stress levels, resulting in telomere erosion in stem cells (Martens and Nawrot 2013).
2. **Impaired telomerase activity:** Telomerase is an enzyme that plays a role in preserving the length of telomeres by appending nucleotide sequences to chromosome ends.

Endocrine-disrupting chemicals (EDCs) can hinder telomerase function, which impairs the capacity of stem cells to uphold their telomeres and results in accelerated aging (Boccardi and Herbig 2012).
3. **Increased cellular senescence:** Shortened telomeres can trigger cellular senescence, a state where cells stop dividing but remain metabolically active. EDCs can thus promote senescence in stem cells by accelerating telomere shortening and impairing telomerase activity, contributing to tissue dysfunction and aging (Franco et al. 2017).
4. **Epigenetic modifications:** Epigenetic changes can be triggered by EDCs and influence how telomeres are regulated in the body's cells. For example, certain EDC exposures have been associated with changes in gene expression related to telomere maintenance, which could affect the function and lifespan of stem cells (Khalil et al. 2018).

Nervous System Effects

Neurodegenerative conditions: Certain environmental chemicals have been linked to diseases like Alzheimer's and Parkinson's that affect the brain and nervous system. Over an extended period of time, their impact on brain function and protein buildup lead to motor impairments. Alzheimer's disease is a condition that affects the brain and memory functions.

1. **Alzheimer's Disease**
    » **Mechanisms of action:** EDCs (endocrine-disrupting chemicals) like pesticides and heavy metals such as lead and mercury can cause stress and neuroinflammation known to contribute to the development of Alzheimer's disease (Bal-Price et al. 2012). These substances have the potential to interfere with the functioning of mitochondria, leading to

the buildup of amyloid beta plaques and tau tangles—the hallmark characteristics of Alzheimer's disease pathology (Bal-Price et al. 2012).
- » **Research findings:** Research studies indicate that being exposed to lead during early development has been connected to levels of amyloid precursor protein and deposition of amyloid beta in the brain as one ages. Likewise, exposure to pesticides has been linked with decreased mental abilities and a greater likelihood of developing Alzheimer's disease (Landrigan et al. 2005).

2. **Parkinson's Disease**
   - » **Mechanisms of action:** Parkinson's disease is a condition that affects movement and can cause tremors, stiffness, and difficulty with balance and coordination. EDCs can contribute to Parkinson's disease by causing harm to mitochondrial function and triggering the accumulation of alpha-synuclein protein in the brain, which forms clumps. Studies have demonstrated how certain pesticides such as paraquat and maneb specifically harm neurons in the substantia nigra region, which is a key characteristic of Parkinson's disease (Tanner et al. 2011).
   - » **Research findings:** Studies have shown that people with exposure to pesticides are at increased risk of developing Parkinson's disease (Tanner et al. 2011). Moreover, when multiple endocrine-disrupting chemicals (EDCs) are combined, the risk is further amplified due to their synergistic effect (Tanner et al. 2011).

Multigenerational Impact

Transgenerational effects: The impact of endocrine-disrupting chemicals (EDCs) can extend across generations through alterations that are passed down to offspring. This phenomenon indicates that the implications of exposure in one generation can influence the well-being of future generations by resulting in fertility complications, metabolic imbalances, and heightened vulnerability to illnesses.

1. **Epigenetic Modifications**
   » The effects of EDCs include changing DNA methylation patterns and modifying histones and noncoding RNA expression to control gene activity without altering the DNA itself. These epigenetic changes can endure across cell generations and impact the health and growth of generations (Skinner 2014). For example, my grandmother may have been exposed to certain chemicals that led to a genetic change that now increases my risk for diabetes and cancer.
   » Chemical substances like bisphenol A (BPA), diethylstilbestrol (DES), and vinclozolin have been proven to have effects across generations. For example, BPA can change genes related to reproductive abilities, resulting in fertility problems for generations (Skinner 2014).

2. **Health Implications**
   » **Reproductive issues:** Offspring of individuals exposed to EDCs may experience reduced fertility, altered puberty timing, and increased susceptibility to reproductive disorders such as polycystic ovary syndrome (PCOS) and testicular dysgenesis syndrome (Manikkam et al. 2012).
   » **Metabolic disorders:** Transgenerational exposure to EDCs may heighten the likelihood of obesity and insulin resistance. They contribute to the development of type 2 diabetes in future generations due to epigenetic modifications affecting metabolic processes (Skinner 2014).

» **Increased disease susceptibility:** EDCs can increase the susceptibility to various diseases including cardiovascular diseases, immune disorders, and cancers across generations. These effects highlight the long-lasting and pervasive impact of EDC exposure on public health (Skinner 2014).

Endocrine-Related Cancers

EDCs can mimic or block hormones like estrogen and testosterone, which are implicated in hormone-sensitive cancers such as breast, prostate, and ovarian cancers. Since the 1970s, there has been an exponential rise in cancers since the introduction of plastics and EDCs. We are now seeing higher rates presenting earlier in our forties and fifties.

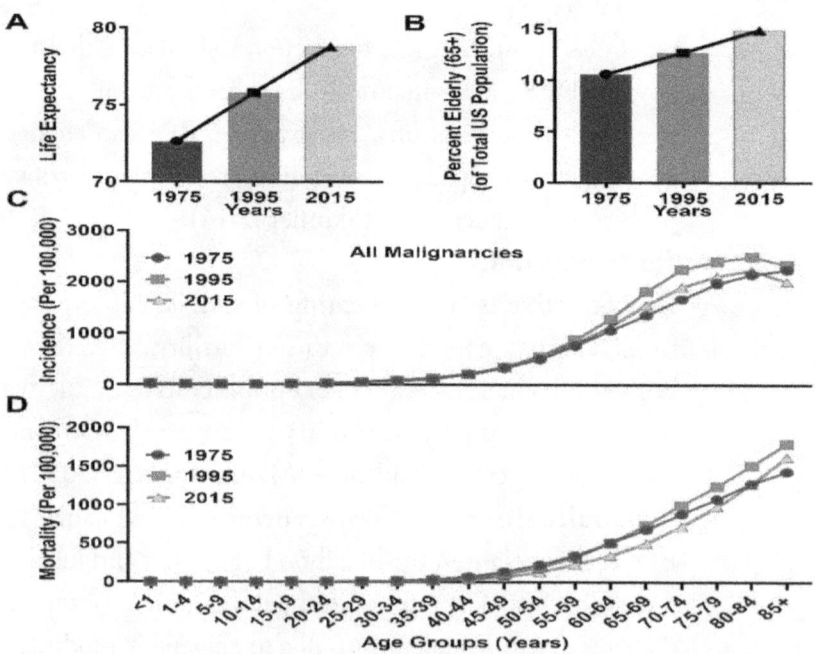

This Photo by Unknown Author is licensed under CC BY

Hormone-Sensitive Cancers
- **Mechanisms of action:** Endocrine-disrupting chemicals (EDCs) can mimic or block hormones like estrogen and testosterone, leading to irregular hormonal pathways needed for the development and progression of hormone-sensitive cancers, including breast, prostate, and ovarian cancers. EDCs can bind to hormone receptors, activate or inhibit signaling pathways, and affect gene expression related to cell growth, apoptosis (cell death), and metastasis (spread of the cancer) (Diamanti-Kandarakis et al. 2009).
- **Breast cancer:** EDCs like bisphenol A (BPA), phthalates, and polychlorinated biphenyls (PCBs) are estrogen mimickers that can bind to the estrogen receptor (ER) and stimulate the proliferation of breast cancer cells. Studies have found that exposure to these chemicals is a risk factor for breast cancer. BPA has been found to increase the growth of ER-positive breast cancer cells and to contribute to tumorigenesis (Vandenberg et al. 2007).
- **Prostate cancer:** As with breast cancer, prostate cancer can be influenced by EDCs via their action at the androgen receptor (AR). Estrogenic chemicals like BPA and certain pesticides can act as androgens or antiandrogens to affect the growth and function of prostate cells. Research has established that EDC exposure is a risk factor for prostate cancer because these chemicals can stimulate the growth of cancer cells and suppress apoptotic processes that lead to tumor growth and progression (Prins et al. 2007).
- **Ovarian cancer:** Estrogenic and antiestrogenic EDCs can also affect the development of ovarian cancer. Phthalates and dioxins are known to affect the ovaries and alter their function, resulting in hormonal imbalances that may predispose to

ovarian cancer. These disturbances can drive the development of cancerous ovary lesions through regulations of cell growth, maturation, and death (Kim et al. 2015).

Cancer Development: Potential Mechanisms of Action

1. **DNA damage:** Oxidative stress induced by EDCs can lead to the modification of the genetic material, namely DNA, which can result in cancer development. Reactive oxygen species (ROS) produced during EDC exposure can lead to genetic instability, which is a characteristic of cancer cells (Soto and Sonnenschein 2010).
2. **Epigenetic modifications:** EDCs can also bring about epigenetic changes, including DNA methylation and histone modifications that can silence or activate genes without changing the DNA sequence. These epigenetic changes can turn off the genes that prevent cancer growth (tumor suppressor genes) and turn on genes that encourage cancer growth (oncogenes) to promote cancer progression (Skinner 2014).
3. **Altered hormone metabolism:** EDCs can act on the enzymes that regulate hormone metabolism, increasing the levels of active hormones that can stimulate the growth of hormone-dependent cancers. For example, some EDCs work by stopping the enzymes that break down estrogens, keeping estrogenic signaling active for longer (Diamanti-Kandarakis et al. 2009).
4. **Inflammatory pathways:** EDC-induced chronic inflammation can lead to a tumor-promoting environment. Cytokines and growth factors that are secreted during the inflammatory response to EDC exposure can stimulate cell growth, angiogenesis, and metastasis (Kim et al. 2015).

Scan to learn more about how cancer develops.

All videos are provided courtesy of Alilia Medical Media. Copying and/or downloading of any of the videos or animations to any social media platforms such as YouTube, Facebook, or TikTok is strictly prohibited.

©Alila Medical Media. All medical materials are for information purposes *only* and are *not* intended to be medical advice.

Reproductive Complications

From infertility and endometriosis in women to low sperm count and quality in men, a number of problems with the reproductive system can be caused by EDCs and may be long-term or even permanent.

Infertility and endometriosis: In women, EDCs can interfere with the normal hormonal balance that is required for proper reproductive performance and may result in infertility or endometriosis. For instance, phthalates are known to interfere with ovarian functions and increase the risk of endometriosis.

Polycystic ovary syndrome (PCOS): Some of the EDCs that have been linked with the development and worsening of PCOS include BPA and phthalates. PCOS is an endocrine disorder that affects women in their childbearing years and is characterized by irregular menstrual cycles, hyperandrogenism (elevated testosterone levels), and polycystic ovaries. These chemicals can affect the endocrine system and thus lead to hormonal imbalances that are characteristic of PCOS (Rutkowska and Rachon 2014).

Low sperm count and quality: In men, EDCs can lead to low sperm production and quality by affecting the production of testosterone and the development of sperm. It has been established that chemicals such as BPA and phthalates are bad for the male reproductive system and may lead to infertility (Hauser et al. 2006).

Metabolic disorders: Increasing evidence suggests that EDC exposure is associated with metabolic disorders including obesity, prediabetes, and diabetes. These chemicals can affect the blood sugar and fat storage of the body and can lead to long-term health complications. More will be discussed in detail in chapter five.

Autoimmune Diseases

Link between EDCs and autoimmune diseases: New research shows that EDCs can cause autoimmune diseases such as rheumatoid arthritis (RA) and systemic lupus erythematosus (SLE). EDCs can affect the immune system and make it overreact or underreact, resulting in the body attacking its own tissues.

1. **Mechanisms of Action**
    - » **Immune system dysregulation:** EDCs such as BPA, dioxins, and phthalates can interfere with the development and function of immune cells. These chemicals can alter cytokine production, skewing immune system

dysregulation. EDCs including BPA, dioxins, and phthalates can affect the growth and function of immune cells. These chemicals can modify cytokine secretion, tilting the immune response toward the pro-inflammatory phenotype which is characteristic of autoimmune diseases (Rogers et al. 2013).

» **Molecular mimicry:** It has been established that some EDCs can cause molecular mimicry in which the immune system attacks the body's own tissues because they resemble foreign antigens. This can lead to the development of autoimmune diseases including RA and SLE (Selmi et al. 2012).

2. **Rheumatoid Arthritis (RA)**
    » **EDCs and RA:** Some EDCs have been found to be related with higher chances of developing RA. For example, phthalates and BPA have been reported to worsen the inflammation that is associated with RA by activating the inflammatory pathways (Rogers et al. 2013).
    » **Research findings:** Studies have shown that people with higher levels of EDC exposure are more likely to develop RA, suggesting that these chemicals may cause the development of autoimmune disease (Pollard et al. 2019).

3. **Systemic Lupus Erythematosus (SLE)**
    » **EDCs and SLE:** EDCs can worsen the immune dysfunction seen in SLE, a systemic inflammatory disease characterized by inflammation and tissue damage. The onset and progression of SLE have been associated with BPA and heavy metals (Selmi et al. 2012).
    » **Research findings:** Epidemiological studies have shown that EDC exposure is related to higher rates of SLE, and

that these chemicals may act as triggers of autoimmune reactions (Cooper et al. 2009).

Mental Health Effects

Studies on the effects of EDCs on mental health have started to emerge, showing that EDC exposure is linked to anxiety, depression, and autism spectrum disorders (ASD). This is an area of research that has only been explored relatively recently, so the results are still quite incomplete.

1. **Mechanisms of Action**
   » **Neurotransmitter disruption:** EDCs can act on the synthesis, release, and function of neurotransmitters that are necessary for normal mental function. Benzaldehyde can act as an endocrine disruptor through the mechanism of BPA and phthalates that can interfere with the serotonergic and dopaminergic pathways and cause mood and cognitive disorders (Braun et al. 2011).
   » **Hormonal imbalance:** EDCs can affect the level of stress hormones like cortisol that can lead to anxiety and depression. These hormonal changes can have a severe impact on the brain and the overall mental health (Patisaul and Bateman 2008).
2. **Anxiety and Depression**
   » **EDCs and mood disorders:** It has been established that exposure to EDCs increases the incidence of anxiety and depression. For example, BPA affects the levels of anxiety and depressive symptoms in both animal and human populations (Harley et al. 2013).

» **Research findings:** The studies showed that children and adults with higher levels of EDCs in their systems are likely to have mood disorders (Braun et al. 2011).
3. **Autism Spectrum Disorders (ASD)**
   » **EDCs and ASD:** There is growing evidence that prenatal and early-life exposure to EDCs may increase the risk of ASD. EDCs can act as brain and neurodevelopmental toxins and cause behavioral and cognitive abnormalities (Kim et al. 2017).
   » **Research findings:** Epidemiological studies have established relationships between maternal exposure to EDCs like phthalates and the risk of ASD in children. These findings are significant as they point to the neurodevelopmental consequences of EDC exposure (Lyall et al. 2017).

Chronic Exposure to EDCs and Hair Loss

Alopecia (hair loss) can be caused by genetic factors, hormonal imbalances, and certain environmental factors. Recent studies show that prolonged exposure to endocrine-disrupting chemicals (EDCs) can also cause hair loss through endocrine and cellular alterations.

Mechanisms of EDC-Induced Hair Loss

1. **Hormonal imbalances:** EDCs affect the endocrine system and result in hormonal imbalances that affect hair growth. For instance, substances like BPA and phthalates can act as estrogens or androgens and thereby alter the function of hair follicles and may lead to hair loss (Meeker et al. 2011).
2. **Disruption of hair follicle cycles:** Hair has growth phases, which include the growth of hair, regression of hair, and rest of hair. EDCs can interfere with these cycles by modifying the hair follicle-signaling pathways. Continued exposure to EDCs

can mean that more hair follicles are in the telogen phase, which can lead to increased hair loss (Thornton et al. 2010).
3. **Oxidative stress and inflammation:** EDCs can cause oxidative stress and inflammation in the scalp, which can damage hair follicles and hamper their ability to produce healthy hair. Dioxins and PCBs are known to enhance the formation of reactive oxygen species (ROS), which are harmful to cells and may lead to hair loss (Sharma et al. 2016).
4. **Impaired microcirculation:** In order to function properly, the scalp needs a sufficient blood supply to transport nutrients and oxygen to the hair follicles. EDCs can harm blood vessels and reduce blood flow to the scalp, which can weaken hair follicles and cause hair loss (Khalil et al. 2018).

Specific EDCs Linked to Hair Loss
1. **Bisphenol A (BPA):** BPA is used in plastics, and it has been found to affect the androgen and estrogen signaling, which can lead to hormonal imbalances that are known to affect hair growth. Studies have indicated that exposure to BPA leads to changes in the hair follicle cycle and increased hair loss (Akinbami et al. 2016).
2. **Phthalates:** Phthalates are used in many consumer products and have been linked with lower levels of sex hormones such as testosterone. This hormonal change can be detrimental to the hair follicles and may lead to hair loss (Meeker et al. 2011).
3. **Polychlorinated biphenyls (PCBs):** PCBs are environmental pollutants that have been found to cause oxidative stress and inflammation in various tissues, including the scalp. It has been established that exposure to PCBs can lead to hair follicle damage and hair loss (Sharma et al. 2016).

4. **Dioxins:** Dioxins are industrial by-products that are very toxic and can cause hormonal imbalance and oxidative stress, which can damage hair follicles and lead to hair loss (Thornton et al. 2010).

Effects of Chlorine, Fluoride, and Heavy Metals on Hair Loss

Chlorine
Chlorine, which is used to kill bacteria in water, can strip the hair and scalp of their natural oils and lead to dry and irritated skin. Repeated contact can cause hair cuticles to be damaged, which makes the hair prone to breaking and increases hair loss. It also has the ability to disturb the microbiome of the scalp, which is not good for hair growth.

Fluoride
Fluoride in water and in dental products has been found to be harmful to the body and has been linked to thyroid problems. Hypothyroidism, a condition that is linked to fluoride, can cause hair loss and thinning. Oxidative stress can also be brought on by fluoride, which will further damage the hair follicles (Chouhan et al. 2017).

Heavy Metals (Lead, Mercury, Arsenic, Cadmium)
These heavy metals can enter the body and affect the body's functions in several ways. These metals can cause oxidative stress, inflammation, and hormonal changes, all of which can lead to hair loss. For instance, the use of lead and cadmium has been linked with hair loss and hair weight reduction (Khanna et al. 2013).

EDCs, Angiogenesis, and Illness
Angiogenesis is the natural formation of new blood vessels from existing ones, which is necessary for growth, development, and wound

healing. It is also used in pathological conditions, including cancer, where angiogenesis can help cancer growth and metastasis. Endocrine-disrupting chemicals (EDCs) have been found to have adverse effects on angiogenesis and may be responsible for several health problems.

Effects of EDCs on Angiogenesis
1. **Enhancement of tumor angiogenesis:** EDCs can boost the angiogenesis of tumors to bolster the growth of cancer. Estrogens such as bisphenol A (BPA) and phthalates have been found to enhance the production of proangiogenic cytokines, including vascular endothelial growth factor (VEGF), to foster tumor vascularization and growth (Ho et al. 2017).
2. **Interference of normal angiogenesis:** In addition to stimulating abnormal angiogenesis, EDCs can also interfere with proper angiogenic control. This can hinder wound healing and tissue repair, and may result in chronic wounds and other complications (Watson et al. 2019).
3. **Epigenetic modifications:** EDCs can lead to epigenetic alterations that can switch on or off the genes regulating angiogenesis. For instance, exposure to certain EDCs has been associated with the hypermethylation of the promoter regions of angiogenesis-related genes, thus silencing them and contributing to the pathogenesis of cardiovascular diseases (Zama and Uzumcu 2010).

Health Implications
1. **Cancer:** As angiogenesis stimulators, EDCs can help in the growth and spread of tumors, and thus, they are a significant issue in oncology. Angiogenesis boosts the ability of tumors to get the necessary nutrients and oxygen for their development and growth.

2. **Cardiovascular diseases:** Altered angiogenesis can also lead to the development of cardiovascular diseases. Inflammation of the inner linings of the arteries (atherosclerosis) and ischemic diseases may occur due to abnormal angiogenesis as it can hinder the formation and regeneration of blood vessels (Ho et al. 2017).
3. **Reproductive health:** EDCs can act on angiogenic processes in reproductive organs, thus affecting fertility and pregnancy. Abnormal angiogenesis in the placenta, for example, can lead to complications such as preeclampsia and a small (for gestational age) fetus (Watson et al. 2019).

Conclusion

EDCs are linked to both short- and long-term health issues with consequences to almost all organ systems and manifestations as acute and chronic diseases. Knowing these risks is the first step to preventing exposure and improving long-term health. As we realize the full effects of their impact, it becomes crucial to address the threats posed by EDCs with immediate effect. This is why there is a need for more research, awareness, and regulatory measures to minimize the effects of these environmental contaminants on the public. The effects of chronic exposure to EDCs include an increased risk of hormone-sensitive cancers of the breast, prostate, and ovaries. The mechanisms by which EDCs contribute to cancer development must be well understood to prevent these risks. To this end, we can advocate for stricter regulations, increase public awareness on avoidance of EDCs, and thus contribute to the fight against these serious diseases.

CHAPTER FIVE:

EDCs and Development of Prediabetes and Type 2 Diabetes

Prediabetes is a condition where the blood glucose level is higher than normal but not high enough to be called diabetes. It is defined as a condition where laboratory tests are positive for fasting blood sugar of more than 100 mg/dl and less than 126 mg/dl or HbA1c of more than 5.6 percent and less than 6.5 percent. It is a well-recognized risk factor for progressing to type 2 diabetes and its complications. There is growing evidence that endocrine-disrupting chemicals (EDCs) can lead to prediabetes.

Mechanisms by Which EDCs Contribute to Prediabetes

1. **Insulin resistance:** To fully understand insulin resistance, let us imagine that your body is a city. In this city, every cell is a house, and sugar (glucose) is the fuel those houses need to stay powered, much like electricity. However, sugar can't just walk in the front door. It needs a key. Insulin is like the trusted delivery driver from the fuel company. Every time you eat, especially carbs, sugar enters your bloodstream. The

pancreas sends out insulin to deliver that sugar to each house (cell). Then insulin (the delivery driver) rings the doorbell and uses its key to unlock the door so sugar can enter and power the house. But let's say you went on an online spending spree and ordered too much sugar. The tons of sugar being delivered every day is more than the houses really need or can handle. In the beginning, insulin keeps up with the demands. But over time, the houses (cells) start getting overwhelmed. They get tired of all the knocking on the door, and eventually, they stop answering the door as quickly. The cells have now become resistant to the action of insulin. EDCs can worsen this process. They can interfere with the insulin-signaling pathways and thus result in insulin resistance that is a prediabetes manifestation. Prolonged usage of insulin results in elevated blood sugar levels. For instance, BPA and phthalates have been seen to interfere with insulin receptor signaling and glucose metabolism by cells (Alonso-Magdalena et al. 2011).

2. **Altered adipogenesis:** EDCs can boost the development of stem cells into adipocytes (fat cells), and this leads to obesity, which is a precursor to prediabetes. Having more fat tissue, especially visceral fat located around your internal organs, can worsen insulin resistance and inflammation that are stepping stones in the development of prediabetes. Some chemicals, including BPA and certain pesticides, have been found to support adipogenesis and enhance fat storage (Grün and Blumberg 2009).

3. **Chronic inflammation:** EDCs can lead to prolonged inflammation, which is a well-known cause of insulin resistance and prediabetes. Adipose tissue produces inflammatory cytokines that can attach to insulin-signaling pathways. Elevated levels of inflammatory markers such as CRP are usually present

in individuals with prediabetes, denoting a state of systemic inflammation (Hotamisligil 2006).
4. **Oxidative stress:** EDCs can enhance the generation of reactive oxygen species (ROS), which can lead to oxidative stress. Oxidative stress generates free radicals that can damage cellular components such as proteins, lipids, and DNA, thus disrupting insulin signaling and pancreatic function. This oxidative damage is one of the factors that leads to the development of insulin resistance and prediabetes (Sargis et al. 2010).
5. **Alteration of the microbiota of the gut:** EDCs can change the composition and function of the good gut bacteria which is involved in metabolic regulation. Dysbiosis, a term used to describe an imbalance in the gut bacteria, can cause increased intestinal permeability, systemic inflammation, and metabolic complications, all of which are risk factors for the development of prediabetes (Claus et al. 2016).

Type 2 diabetes mellitus (T2DM) is a metabolic disorder characterized by high blood glucose due to insulin resistance and impaired insulin secretion. The diagnosis of diabetes is made when your fasting glucose is more than 126 mg/dl, random nonfasting glucose is more than 200 mg/dl, or HbA1c is more than 6.5 percent. Increasing evidence suggests that endocrine-disrupting chemicals (EDCs) are important factors leading to the development of T2DM. These chemicals that are available in the environment can act on the endocrine system and other metabolic functions and may contribute to the onset of diabetes with increasing incidence over the years. As you can see in the diagram below, the rates of obesity and diabetes have been rapidly increasing and correlate with the increased use of plastics. Since the 1980s, we have seen a 10 percent increase in diabetes. That is equivalent to nearly 4 million people. It is estimated that there are currently 38 million Americans with diabetes. Although there are many factors such as poor diet, sedentary lifestyle, and socioeconomic reasons for the increasing rates of diabetes, we cannot ignore the impact of EDCs on this worrisome trajectory.

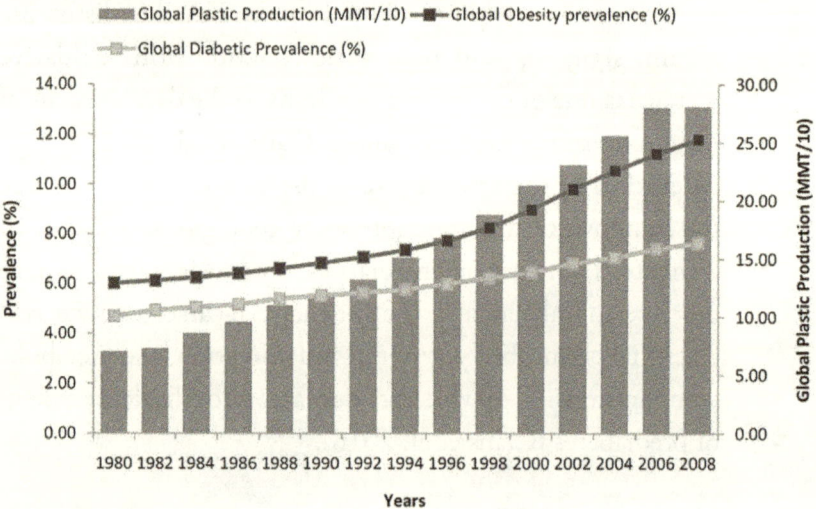

This Photo by Unknown Author is licensed under CC BY

Understanding Type 2 Diabetes Mellitus

T2DM develops when the body's cells become resistant to the effects of insulin, a hormone produced by the pancreas that regulates blood glucose levels. Over time, the pancreas cannot produce enough insulin to overcome this resistance, leading to hyperglycemia (high blood sugar). Risk factors for T2DM include genetics, obesity, physical inactivity, and now, exposure to EDCs.

Below is a summary of insulin action. In the brain, insulin helps regulate appetite and satiety by acting on the hypothalamus. It also signals the brain that the body has enough energy, helping to suppress hunger. The liver is a major site for glucose storage and production. Insulin inhibits gluconeogenesis (the production of glucose) and promotes glycogen synthesis (the storage of glucose for later use). The muscle is the main consumer of blood glucose, especially after eating. Insulin stimulates glucose uptake into muscle cells via GLUT4 transporters and promotes glycogen storage and protein synthesis. The adipose (fat) tissues store energy and regulate metabolism. Insulin promotes fat storage by encouraging the uptake of glucose and the conversion to triglycerides and inhibits lipolysis (the breakdown of stored fat).

However, when there is insulin resistance, the opposite actions occur. We may see increased appetite, cravings, and risk of developing neurodegenerative diseases like Alzheimer's disease (sometimes called type 3 diabetes). The liver keeps producing glucose even when it isn't needed, contributing to high blood sugar levels. Cholesterol and inflammation build up, leading to fatty liver disease. The muscles become less responsive to insulin, reducing glucose uptake and contributing to fatigue due to mitochondrial dysfunction and high blood sugar. Lastly, fat cells become inflamed and dysfunctional, increasing fat accumulation and contributing to obesity and metabolic inflammation.

TOXIC OVERLOAD: The Invisible Endocrine-Disrupting Chemicals Making Us Sick, Fat, and Tired

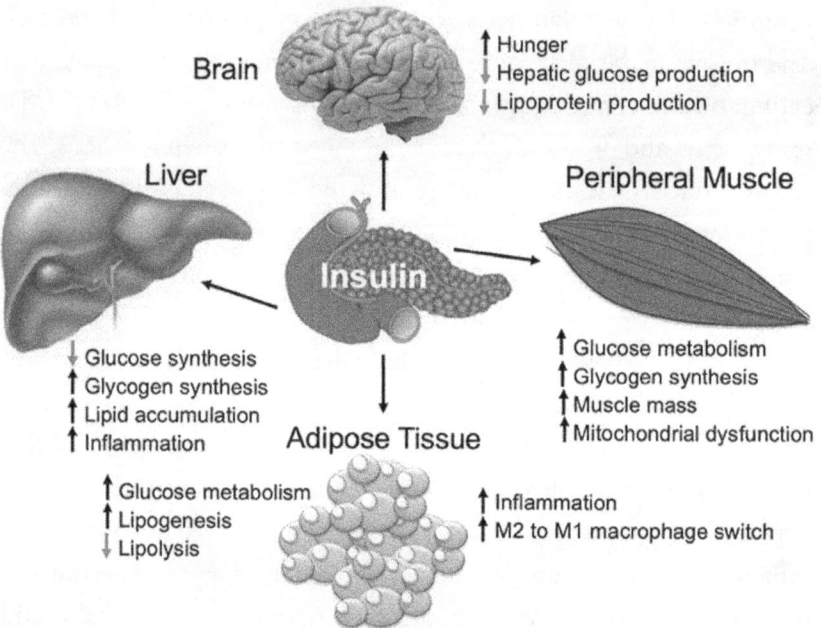

This Photo by Unknown Author is licensed under CC BY

Scan to learn more about diabetes.

All videos are provided courtesy of Alilia Medical Media. Copying and/or downloading of any of the videos or animations to any social media platforms such as YouTube, Facebook, or TikTok is strictly prohibited.

©Alila Medical Media. All medical materials are for information purposes *only* and are *not* intended to be medical advice.

How EDCs Contribute to Type 2 Diabetes

1. **Insulin resistance:** EDCs can interfere with the insulin-signaling pathways and thus lead to insulin resistance. Chemicals like BPA and phthalates have been found to interfere with the function of insulin receptors on the cell surface, thus preventing the cells from absorbing glucose from the bloodstream (Alonso-Magdalena et al. 2011).
2. **Impaired insulin secretion:** EDCs also affect the pancreatic beta cells that produce insulin. It has been established that exposure to certain EDCs can result in beta cell damage and a reduction in the secretion of insulin in response to blood glucose concentrations (García-Arevalo et al. 2014).
3. **Altered adipogenesis:** EDCs can also stimulate the differentiation of stem cells into adipocytes (fat cells), thus adding to the problem of obesity, which is a significant cause of type 2 diabetes mellitus (T2DM). More fat tissue only worsens insulin resistance and inflammation, and thus increases the risk of diabetes (Grün and Blumberg 2009).
4. **Chronic inflammation:** EDCs can also bring about low-grade chronic inflammation, which is a central mediator of insulin resistance. The inflammatory cytokines secreted by adipose tissue can act on insulin receptors and thereby participate in the pathogenesis of T2DM (Thayer et al. 2012).

Scientific Evidence
1. **Bisphenol A (BPA):** BPA is a plasticizer and has been studied extensively in relation to metabolic disorders. Numerous studies have established that exposure to BPA is linked with heightened insulin resistance and raised fasting glucose concentrations, both of which are risk factors for T2DM (Alonso-Magdalena et al. 2011).
2. **Phthalates:** Phthalates are used in many consumer products and are related to metabolic disturbances. Research has indicated that higher levels of phthalate metabolites in the urine are associated with increased waist circumference and insulin resistance, thus implying a role in the development of T2DM (Svensson et al. 2011).
3. **Persistent organic pollutants (POPs):** POPs are environmental contaminants that include dioxins and polychlorinated biphenyls (PCBs) and are environmentally persistent and bioaccumulated in human tissues. Epidemiological studies have indicated that exposure to POPs is a risk factor for T2DM, possibly through its impact on insulin signaling and glucose metabolism (Lee et al. 2010).

Mechanisms of Action
1. **Hormonal disruption:** EDCs can act as hormone agonists (stimulators) or antagonists (blockers), and therefore, interfere with the endocrine system. This hormonal change can lead to glucose and lipid metabolic disorders, which can lead to insulin resistance and T2DM.
2. **Epigenetic modifications:** EDCs can also bring about epigenetic changes that lead to heritable changes in gene expression without a change in the DNA sequence. These changes can affect genes that control glucose metabolism and

insulin signaling and can lead to the development of T2DM (Janesick and Blumberg, 2011).
3. **Oxidative stress:** EDCs can enhance the generation of reactive oxygen species (ROS) and result in oxidative stress. Oxidative stress can damage cells and tissues, which in turn, can lead to insulin signaling and pancreatic dysfunction and the progression to T2DM (Sargis et al. 2010).

Strategies for Reducing the Impact of EDCs

1. **Regulatory measures:** This can be done by strict enforcement of policies that limit the use and discharge of EDCs. It is also important to have policies that aim at minimizing EDC pollution in food, water, and consumer products.
2. **Public awareness:** This can be achieved through community education on the sources and effects of EDCs. People will be in a better position to make the right decisions and avoid being exposed to these chemicals as a result of being informed. The campaigns can also be based on the theme of using EDC-free products and following better dietary guidelines.
3. **Research and innovation:** The importance of this cannot be overemphasized, as more knowledge is gained about the ways in which EDCs affect the body and health. The search for new and safer alternatives to EDCs, and new methods of detecting and eliminating these chemicals in the environment, will minimize risks to health.

Conclusion

The reviewed articles show that EDCs lead to the development of prediabetes through insulin resistance, altered adipogenesis, chronic inflammation, oxidative stress, and disruption of the gut microbiota. This knowledge is important in the development of strategies that can be used to prevent or lessen the adverse health consequences of EDC exposure. More research, awareness, and regulations are needed to ensure that the general public is protected from these environmental pollutants.

The evidence that has been presented in this chapter shows that EDCs are major contributors to the incidence of type 2 diabetes mellitus and that effective control measures are therefore necessary. As we learn more about the ways that EDCs interfere with metabolic functions, we can design more specific strategies for prevention and treatment of T2DM. Through policy, public outreach, and scientific endeavors, it is possible to lessen the impact of EDCs and improve the quality of life for future generations.

CHAPTER SIX:

The Relationship Between EDCs and the Development of Thyroid Disease

The thyroid gland helps in metabolism, growth, and development through production of thyroid hormones. Endocrine-disrupting chemicals (EDCs) can alter the thyroid function and lead to different thyroid diseases, including thyroid nodules. This chapter describes how EDCs influence the thyroid gland and discusses the resulting thyroid pathologies.

Mechanisms of EDC Action on the Thyroid

1. **Interruption of hormone production:** EDCs can disrupt the uptake of iodine, a crucial component for thyroid hormone production, by affecting the sodium-iodide symporter. The sodium-iodide symporter is a protein that plays a crucial role in thyroid hormone synthesis and is found in tissue like salivary glands. It functions by transporting iodide ions into cells in the thyroid gland as the first step in producing

thyroid hormones. Some EDCs can mimic or block the action of thyroid-stimulating hormone (TSH), further impacting thyroid hormone synthesis. EDCs can stop the formation of thyroid hormones by disabling thyroid peroxidase (TPO), an enzyme that is required for the formation of thyroxine (T4) and triiodothyronine (T3). For example, PCBs and perchlorate are known to decrease TPO activity, thus decreasing the formation of hormones (Pearce and Braverman 2009). Halogenated chemicals such as fluoride, bromine, and chloride have been known to interfere with the iodination of thyroid hormones.

2. **Alteration of hormone transport:** EDCs can compete with thyroid hormone transport proteins like thyroxine-binding globulin (TBG), and hence, reduce the availability of free hormones to be taken up by the cells. Chemicals such as bisphenol A (BPA), PFAS, perchlorate, and phthalates have been reported to alter the binding of thyroid hormones to their transport proteins, thus reducing the availability of free T4 and T3 (Meeker et al. 2011).

3. **Alteration of hormone metabolism:** EDCs can act on the thyroid hormone metabolism through the modulation of deiodinases, enzymes that convert T4 to the more active T3. Some can increase the clearance rate of thyroid hormone from the body, potentially lowering circulating thyroid hormone levels. Flame retardants such as polybrominated diphenyl ethers (PBDEs) can affect the deiodinase, thus altering the thyroid hormone levels (Butt et al. 2011).

4. **Thyroid receptor antagonism:** Some EDCs are thyroid hormone receptor antagonists and therefore compete with the hormones to attach to the receptors and induce fake signaling. This can result in thyroid hormone resistance and subsequent metabolic dysregulation (Boas et al. 2012). PCBs can disrupt thyroid hormone signaling and affect brain development.

Below is an analysis of the diseases of the thyroid which are connected with EDC exposure.
1. **Hypothyroidism:** Hypothyroidism is a lack of functional thyroid hormones and may be caused by EDCs affecting hormone synthesis, transport, or metabolism. Symptoms of hypothyroidism include lethargy, weight gain, cold sensitivity, and depression (Pearce and Braverman 2009).
2. **Hyperthyroidism:** Hyperthyroidism, the opposite of hypothyroidism, is not as commonly associated with EDCs. Some substances can cause the thyroid to secrete or produce thyroid hormones, leading to symptoms of weight loss, increased heat tolerance, nervousness, and rapid heart rate (Boas et al. 2012).
3. **Autoimmune thyroid diseases:** Evidence suggests that EDCs can cause autoimmune thyroid diseases, including Hashimoto's thyroiditis and Graves' disease. These conditions are characterized by the production of abnormal immune responses to thyroid tissue, which results in chronic inflammation and dysfunction. BPA and other EDCs can affect the immune system and may act as triggers for autoimmune responses (Zoeller et al. 2007).
4. **Thyroid cancer:** Some EDCs like PBDEs and PCBs are known to be associated with thyroid cancer due to long-term exposure. These chemicals can bring about genetic and epigenetic alterations in thyroid cells, which can lead to carcinogenesis. These EDCs have been found to be at higher levels in individuals with thyroid cancer (Miyake et al. 2006).
5. **Thyroid nodules:** Thyroid nodules are benign or malignant lumps in the thyroid gland and can be single or multiple. EDCs can cause thyroid nodules by altering the normal thyroid cell function and promoting abnormal cell growth. BPA and phthalates have been found to induce changes on

the cellular level that can lead to nodule development. These chemicals induce thyroid cell proliferation and may cause nodule formation if exposure is prolonged. A review of the literature found that chronic exposure to these chemicals can lead to the development of thyroid nodules (Lee et al. 2012).

Triclosan and Thyroid Disease

Triclosan is an antimicrobial agent that is used in many household and personal care products, including soaps, toothpastes, and cleaners. Research has been conducted on triclosan and thyroid dysfunction. It has been established that triclosan can act as an endocrine disruptor by interfering with thyroid hormone synthesis and metabolism. Triclosan has been reported to decrease T4 and T3 levels, which may lead to hypothyroidism and other thyroid-related problems (Paul et al. 2010). Because of these concerns and its potential impact on thyroid health, triclosan has been removed from most consumer products after the FDA banned it in 2016.

Conclusion

The impact of EDCs on thyroid function is significant and multifaceted, leading to various thyroid diseases, including thyroid nodules. The case of triclosan illustrates how regulatory measures can mitigate risks associated with EDCs. Understanding these mechanisms and their health implications is crucial for developing effective strategies to protect public health. By raising awareness, advocating for stricter regulations, and reducing exposure to EDCs, we can mitigate their adverse effects on thyroid health and promote overall well-being.

The next chapter will focus specifically on the role of EDCs as "obesogens," exploring their impact on metabolism and weight gain, an increasingly prevalent issue in today's world.

CHAPTER SEVEN:

How EDCs Are Making Us Fat: Their Role as Obesogens

We have explored the impacts of EDCs on a number of health dimensions. But now, we turn to one regard that is emerging as an important part of the modern health dilemma: obesity. Are these omnipresent chemicals causing us to tip the scales in the wrong direction? In this chapter, we will examine EDCs as "obesogens"—substances that may play a role in the obesity epidemic. We will discuss the impact of EDCs on metabolism and obesity.

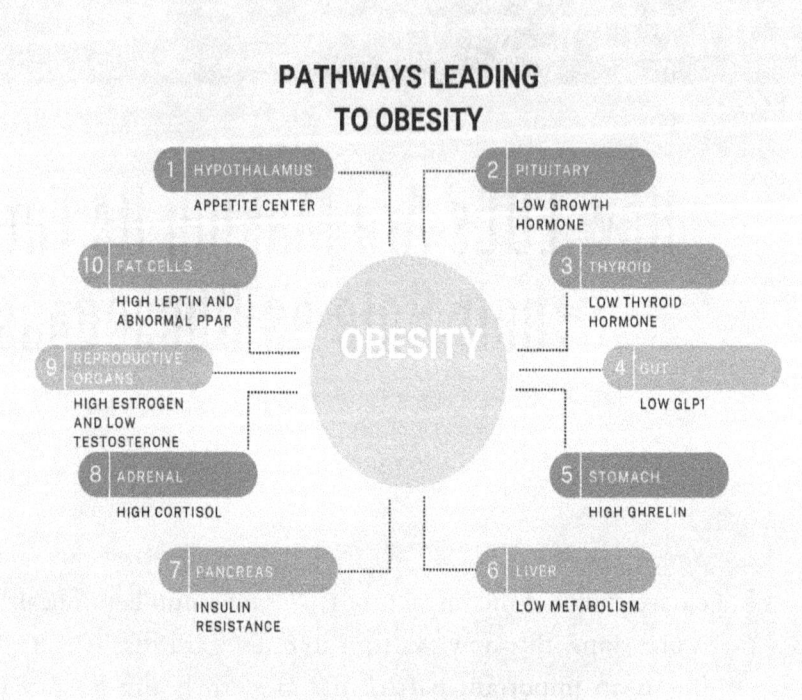

Metabolism: The Body's Engine

The term "metabolism" encompasses the chemical reactions in cells that convert food into energy. It is governed by hormones like insulin, thyroid hormones, and cortisol, making it highly susceptible to endocrine disruption. We need to rethink how we perceive weight gain. It is not as simple as the saying, "too many calories in, and not enough out." It is not just because you are not exercising enough. Weight gain is a symptom of a much bigger issue. Whenever I see a patient for a consult about weight gain, I do my best to screen and rule out possible endocrine disorders such as insulin resistance, thyroid disease, and Cushing's disease (a condition that produces too much cortisol). But the great majority of cases are due to inflammation. Even if you are on the strictest diet and exercise regimen, if you have inflammation, you will struggle to lose weight. The ultimate question is which came first? The inflammation or the obesity? It's the same "did the chicken or egg come first" dilemma. Research has linked higher levels of CRP, a marker of inflammation, with greater weight gain (Tuomisto et al. 2019). The fact is that both coexist, and if we can target the source or root of inflammation, we can achieve more success at combating weight gain. This inflammation appears to be induced by EDCs that further result in hormonal and metabolic alterations.

Obesogens: These new hidden culprits can affect various hormone pathways as shown, leading to weight gain. The term "obesogen" was used to describe chemicals with the potential of promoting weight gain and obesity through metabolic process interference in several ways. The EDCs most often linked with weight gain are DDT, bisphenols (BPA), phthalates, PFAS, dioxin, polychlorinated biphenyls (PCBs), MSG, food preservatives, and tributyl tin which are unfortunately ubiquitous in our air, food, water, clothing, furniture, and personal care products. It is hypothesized that these toxins can change the "set points" of how much food intake results in weight gain and how much exercise is needed to burn it. They are thought to affect how the body stores and uses fat. BPA and flame retardants have been known to increase food consumption. BPA and the others listed above can cause weight disturbances through other pathways such as increasing inflammation, insulin resistance, altering the gut microbiome, and creating dysfunctional fat cells. Other obesogens are phthalates, food additives (such as preservatives and artificial sweeteners), and certain pesticides (like atrazine and glyphosate). Pesticides are commonly found on nonorganic fruits, vegetables, corn, wheat, and rice. I will now explain ten known potential pathways to obesity and weight gain.

1. Hypothalamus

The hypothalamus is the part of the brain that is involved in the regulation of appetite, energy, and metabolism. Endocrine-disrupting chemicals (EDCs) can affect the hypothalamic control of these processes and cause metabolic diseases such as obesity and diabetes.

Mechanisms of EDC Action on the Hypothalamus
- **Disruption of hypothalamic neurons:** These chemicals can impact the neurons, also known as nerve cells, in the hypothalamus that control hunger and satisfaction. The hypothalamus can be affected by chemicals like BPA and phthalates to alter the function of these neurons that regulate appetite and energy balance (Patisaul and Bateman 2008).
- **Alteration of hormone signaling:** Leptin (the "feel full" hormone) and ghrelin (the hunger hormone) are two hormones that are involved in the regulation of appetite and are active in the hypothalamus. EDCs can affect the secretion and action of these hormones, which can lead to increased food intake and decreased energy expenditure. For example, BPA has been found to interfere with leptin signaling and lead to leptin resistance and subsequent weight gain (Rubin 2011). Have you ever wondered why you still feel hungry after eating a healthy portion of food? The imbalance of leptin and ghrelin caused by EDCs could be to blame.
- **Inflammation and oxidative stress:** EDCs can cause inflammation and oxidative stress in the hypothalamus, which can damage neurons and their functions. This can lead to the wrong control of appetite and increase the risk of obesity. Inflammatory cytokines that are produced in response to EDC exposure can interfere with the normal signaling of appetite stimulatory and inhibitory hormones (Thaler et al. 2012).

Effects on Appetite and Metabolism
- **Increased appetite and weight gain:** By disrupting hypothalamic function, EDCs can increase appetite and food intake. This is often accompanied by lower energy expenditure, which leads to weight gain and obesity. It has been found that exposure to EDCs like BPA and phthalates is linked with higher BMI and obesity rates (Newbold et al. 2009).
- **Development of metabolic disorders:** Long-term consumption of EDCs can lead to the growth of metabolic diseases like insulin resistance and type 2 diabetes. The mechanisms of appetite and energy balance disturbed by EDCs can bring about metabolic syndrome—a collection of conditions which are characterized by high blood pressure, high blood sugar, excess fat around the waist, and abnormal cholesterol levels (Heindel and Vandenberg 2015).

2. Pituitary Gland

The pituitary gland, often referred to as the "master gland," plays a pivotal role in regulating various hormones, including growth hormone (GH). Growth hormone is crucial for growth, metabolism, and body composition. It affects energy levels and the rate at which the body burns calories. Low growth hormone levels can lead to fat accumulation. Endocrine-disrupting chemicals (EDCs) can interfere with pituitary function and GH regulation, contributing to weight gain and metabolic disorders.

Mechanisms of EDC Action on the Pituitary Gland
- **Disruption of hormone secretion:** EDCs like BPA, phthalates, and PCBs affect the secretion of GH from the pituitary gland. These chemicals can interfere with the secretory pathways that control the release of GH hormone, resulting in

either high or low levels of the hormone (Diamanti-Kandarakis et al. 2009).
- **Interference with feedback mechanisms:** The hypothalamic-pituitary axis is a negative feedback system that is very intricate and is important in the regulation of hormone secretion. The feedback mechanisms can be disrupted by EDCs that can alter the balance of the hormones that regulate the secretion of GH. For instance, EDCs can affect the neurosecretion of growth hormone-releasing hormone (GHRH) from the hypothalamus, which in turn affects the GH levels (Schug et al. 2011).
- **Direct effects on pituitary cells:** EDCs can have direct cytotoxic (damaging or killing) effects on pituitary cells, impairing their ability to produce and secrete GH. Studies have shown that some exposure to certain EDCs can lead to apoptosis (cell death) or functional changes in the pituitary gland, thus reducing GH output (Wada et al. 2007).

Effects on Growth Hormone and Weight Gain
- **Altered growth hormone levels:** EDCs can lead to dysregulated GH levels, which in turn affects growth and metabolism. Low GH levels are connected with obesity, adiposity, low muscle mass, and metabolic complications. However, high GH levels result in insulin resistance and other metabolic changes (Giustina et al. 2008).
- **Increased fat accumulation:** GH is essential in the process of lipolysis, the breakdown of fat. When EDCs affect and lower the levels of GH, they can inhibit the process of lipolysis, leading to increased fat storage and weight gain, especially around the abdominal region (Giustina et al. 2008).

- **Metabolic syndrome:** The disturbance of GH levels by EDCs can predispose one to metabolic syndrome, which is a collection of conditions that include obesity, insulin resistance, hypertension, and dyslipidemia. Metabolic syndrome is associated with increased risk of developing cardiovascular diseases and type 2 diabetes (Heindel and Vandenberg 2015).

3. Thyroid Gland

EDCs can decrease the production of thyroid hormones by directly affecting the thyroid gland. With reduced thyroid hormone levels, the body's metabolism slows down, making weight gain more likely.

It would be impossible to discuss the general impact of endocrine-disrupting chemicals (EDCs) on our health without referring to their impact on the thyroid gland, the master controller of metabolism and weight. The effects of EDCs on the thyroid gland are rather silent but very damaging in their consequences. These chemicals can interfere with thyroid hormone synthesis, transport, and action, which results in several metabolic complications, including weight gain or loss.

- **Hormone Transportation Roadblocks**
  » Thyroid hormones are carried by the blood to the tissues of the body where they are required. As they flow through the bloodstream, they are paired with proteins like thyroid hormone binding globulin (TBG) and transthyretin (TTR) which act like bodyguards for thyroid hormones to help get them to their desired destinations. EDCs can disrupt the binding of thyroid hormones to these transport proteins. EDCs can attach to the proteins that carry these hormones and make them unavailable or less effective at the target cells.

- **Receptor Binding Disruption**
  » Some EDCs can function as thyroid hormone agonists (activators) or antagonists (blockers) and compete with the hormones for the receptor binding. This likeness or inhibition of metabolic functions can make it difficult to achieve and maintain a healthy body weight.
- **Hypothyroidism and Weight Gain**
  » Hypothyroidism is an autoimmune condition that results in reduced secretion of thyroid hormones and is a common cause of weight gain due to a slowed-down metabolism. Thyroid function can be altered by EDCs, thus causing symptoms similar to those of hypothyroidism.
- **Energy Imbalance**
  » When thyroid function is abnormal, there can be a problem with energy balance in the body. Even if you are consuming the same number of calories, you may gain weight because your body will burn fewer calories.

4. Gut (Small Intestines)

The gastrointestinal tract is also involved in the regulation of metabolism through the secretion of hormones that control hunger and energy utilization. One such hormone is glucagon-like peptide-1 (GLP-1), which has a role in increasing satiety (or the sense of feeling full) and in stimulating insulin secretion. It is the key target hormone of the popular weight loss drugs Ozempic and Wegovy. The adverse effects of EDCs on the gut can lead to reduced production of GLP-1, which in turn results in weight gain and metabolic diseases. Other gut hormones affected by EDCs are GIP and peptide YY.

Glucagon-Like Peptide-1 (GLP-1)

Glucagon-like peptide-1 (GLP-1) is a peripheral hormone that is secreted by L cells in the latter part of the duodenum and jejunum of the small intestine after the ingestion of food (especially carbohydrates). GLP-1 has several important roles in the regulation of glucose and the control of food intake.

How Does GLP-1 Affect Weight?

- **Appetite suppression:** GLP-1 works through the hypothalamus to induce a sense of fullness and thus reduces the desire to eat. When you eat and food enters the small intestine, the L cells make GLP-1 that then sends a message to the appetite center to say, "OK, we've had enough to eat. Please switch the hunger mode to full."
- **Insulin secretion:** GLP-1 acts on the pancreas to secrete insulin in a manner that is dependent on the level of glucose in the blood. This has a role in the improvement of insulin management of blood glucose and may also affect fat metabolism. This makes it an effective way to treat diabetes and even reverse fatty liver disease.
- **Impact on weight:** GLP-1 is involved in weight management due to its role in increasing satiety (feeling full) and controlling blood glucose. Increased levels of GLP-1 are associated with decreased hunger, and therefore decreased food intake, which can be useful in weight loss campaigns.
- **Mechanisms of EDC Action on the Gut and GLP-1**
  - » **Disruption of gut microbiota:** Some EDCs—including BPA, phthalates, and pesticides—can alter the composition and function of the gut microbiota. A healthy gut microbiome is important in the production of GLP-1. This, in turn, results in impaired synthesis and secretion

of GLP-1, which leads to decreased satiety and increased food intake (Claus et al. 2016).

» **Inflammation and oxidative stress:** EDCs can cause inflammation and oxidative stress in the gut, which can lead to the damage of the intestinal lining and the enteroendocrine cells that secrete GLP-1. Thus, chronic inflammation can interfere with the ability of the gut to recognize nutrient signals and decrease GLP-1 production that results in weight gain (Rosenfeld 2017).

» **Direct effects on enteroendocrine cells:** Enteroendocrine cells are specialized cells found in the gastrointestinal tract that produce and secrete hormones involved in digestion, metabolism, and appetite regulation. EDCs can have a direct cytotoxic effect on enteroendocrine cells, which are responsible for the production of GLP-1. These chemicals, including BPA, have been found to reduce the viability and function of these cells, which will result in decreased GLP-1 secretion and subsequent metabolic dysregulation (Ruhlen et al. 2011). One study has linked monosodium glutamate (MSG) with decreased secretion of GLP-1 and disruption of its receptor, which led to increased body mass index and higher prevalence of metabolic syndrome (Shannon et al. 2017).

Effects on GLP-1 and Weight Gain
Reduced satiety and increased appetite: Lower GLP-1 levels lead to decreased satiety and, therefore, to increased food intake and weight gain. Under normal conditions, GLP-1 acts on the brain to induce fullness and decrease appetite. Thus, the reviewed EDC-induced reductions in GLP-1 signaling are thought to make people eat more (Gribble and Reimann 2016).

Impaired insulin secretion: GLP-1 stimulates insulin release during meal intake to regulate blood glucose. Lower GLP-1 levels brought on by EDC exposure can slow this insulinotropic action and may enhance blood glucose levels, leading to increased fat storage and insulin resistance (Holst 2007).

Increased fat accumulation: GLP-1 has been shown to have the properties of enhancing fat oxidation and reducing fat accumulation. Reduced levels of GLP-1 have been found to enhance fat storage, especially in the abdominal region, thus escalating obesity and metabolic syndrome (Drucker 2005).

Glucose-Dependent Insulinotropic Polypeptide (GIP)

Glucose-dependent insulinotropic polypeptide (GIP) is another incretin hormone produced by K cells in the upper part of the small intestine (duodenum and jejunum) following the ingestion of nutrients, especially fats and carbohydrates. It has a crucial role in glucose homeostasis and fat metabolism. GIP accelerates insulin release in response to food intake, especially carbohydrates and fats. It, combined with GLP-1, are the target hormones for the drugs Mounjaro and Zepbound. However, the role it plays in fat storage has been seen to make it contribute to obesity. Endocrine-disrupting chemicals can interact with GIP receptors and contribute to obesity in various ways.

How Does GIP Affect Weight?

- **Insulin secretion:** GIP and GLP-1 work in a similar manner to enhance insulin secretion from the pancreas after food intake to regulate blood glucose levels. However, the effects on metabolism and fat storage are more complicated.
- **Fat storage:** Studies have established that GIP is an anabolic (building up) hormone that enhances fat storage by increasing lipogenesis and suppressing lipolysis, especially in response to

high-fat diets. For this reason, GIP is considered to be one of the most important factors in the pathogenesis of obesity since it regulates fat storage.

- **The effect of weight on various factors:** High levels of GIP have been linked with the increase in fat accumulation, especially in adipose tissue, which can lead to weight gain and obesity. Furthermore, the role of GIP in insulin secretion and fat storage is linked with the metabolic disturbances that are seen in obesity.

Mechanisms of EDC Action on GIP and Obesity

Obesity is a complex metabolic and endocrine disorder that has been associated with exposure to EDCs. There are several proposed ways this can happen. It is probable that more than one defect can exist, making it increasingly difficult for us to lose weight. Scientific research is ongoing to address these concerns.

1. **Disruption of GIP Secretion**
   » EDCs such as bisphenol A (BPA) and phthalates can interfere with the secretion of GIP from K cells in the intestine. These chemicals can alter the secretion of gut hormones, including GIP, which can alter glucose metabolism and promote fat storage (Grün and Blumberg 2009).
2. **Impact on GIP Receptor Signaling**
   » EDCs can alter the sensitivity of GIP receptors on pancreatic beta cells, which are responsible for insulin secretion. This alteration can lead to dysregulated insulin release, contributing to hyperinsulinemia, a condition characterized by excessive insulin levels. Hyperinsulinemia is strongly associated with increased fat storage and obesity (Blumberg 2011).

3. **Promotion of Adipogenesis**
   » We previously reviewed that GIP promotes adipogenesis and lipogenesis in adipose tissue. Therefore, EDCs that increase the level of GIP or the effectiveness of GIP can contribute to the accumulation of fat. It has been established that GIP is able to increase the uptake of fatty acids by adipocytes and to induce the differentiation of preadipocytes into adipocytes. In other words, we can see increased numbers and sizes of fat cells, as well as increased inflammatory fat cells (Miyawaki et al. 2002).
4. **Interaction with Other Hormonal Pathways**
   » EDCs can affect the levels of other hormones such as insulin and glucagon-like peptide-1 (GLP-1) that are involved in the regulation of energy balance, together with GIP. This can only worsen the effects of GIP in causing obesity and lead to increased incidence of weight gain and metabolic complications (Heindel and Blumberg 2019).
5. **Increased Fat Storage**
   » The interaction between EDCs and GIP can lead to increased fat storage, particularly in visceral fat deposits. This effect is compounded by EDC-induced insulin resistance, which impairs the body's ability to effectively utilize glucose, resulting in its storage as fat (Blumberg 2011).
6. **Impaired Glucose Tolerance**
   » Disrupted GIP signaling due to EDC exposure can lead to impaired glucose tolerance, a precursor to type 2 diabetes. As a result, glucose metabolism is compromised and the body starts producing more insulin to utilize the glucose, which leads to fat storage and weight gain (Grün and Blumberg 2009).

7. **Link to Metabolic Syndrome**
   » Chronic exposure to EDCs that affects GIP can contribute to the development of metabolic syndrome, a cluster of conditions that includes obesity, insulin resistance, hypertension, and dyslipidemia. Metabolic syndrome significantly increases the risk of cardiovascular disease and type 2 diabetes (Heindel and Blumberg 2019).

Peptide YY (PYY)

Peptide YY (PYY) is a gut hormone secreted by L cells in the ileum and colon after eating especially with foods containing fiber and protein. PYY is involved in weight regulation through reducing appetite and food intake. PYY levels can be altered, resulting in overeating and obesity. Endocrine-disrupting chemicals (EDCs) can act on PYY secretion and function, thereby affecting the balance of appetite and weight gain.

How Does PYY Affect Weight?
- **Appetite regulation:** PYY works in the brain, particularly the hypothalamus, to suppress hunger and increase the feeling of fullness. It is secreted according to the number of calories in the food, where more calories result in more PYY being released.
- **Gastric emptying:** PYY decreases gastric emptying, meaning that food remains in the stomach for a longer period of time, thus leading to fullness and reduced food intake.
- **Impact on weight:** Enhanced PYY levels are associated with suppressed appetite, and thus reduced food intake, which is beneficial for weight management. Abnormalities in PYY, whether through underproduction or nonfunctioning receptors, can cause increased hunger, overeating, and obesity.

Mechanisms of EDC Action on PYY and Obesity
1. **Disruption of PYY Secretion**
   » Much like BPA and phthalates, other environmental contaminants can interfere with the secretion of PYY from the gut. These chemicals can interact with the enteroendocrine cells that secrete PYY and lead to a decreased secretion of this hormone after food intake (Grün and Blumberg 2009).
2. **Interference with PYY Receptor Signaling**
   » PYY exerts its effects by binding to receptors (for example, the Y2 receptor) for in the brain and gastrointestinal tract. EDCs can act on the PYY's signaling pathways that mediate its action on these receptors, and thus decreases its efficiency in suppressing appetite and food intake. This disruption may lead to enhanced appetite and overeating (Heindel and Blumberg 2019).
3. **Impact on Gut Microbiota**
   » EDCs can alter the composition of the gut microbiota, which is involved in the regulation of gut hormones such as PYY. The imbalance in the gut microbiota (dysbiosis) induced by EDCs can also affect PYY secretion, adding to the problems of appetite dysregulation and weight gain (Janesick and Blumberg 2016).

Effects on PYY and Weight Gain
1. **Reduced Satiety and Increased Appetite**
   » Exposure to EDCs can lead to reduced PYY levels, which in turn leads to reduced satiety and increased appetite and food intake. PYY is supposed to tell the hypothalamus that it is full after a meal. When PYY production or signal transduction is downregulated, a person may keep

on eating and even gain weight (Janesick and Blumberg 2016).

2. **Contribution to Obesity**
   » Long-term exposure to EDCs that affect PYY function may be linked to the development of obesity. The desynchronization of the satiety signals may lead to overeating, increased fat storage, and increased tendency to gain weight, especially in an environment where there is a lot of food that is high in calories and low in nutrients (Grün & Blumberg 2009).

3. **Metabolic Implications**
   » Aside from its role in appetite control, PYY is also involved in the regulation of glucose metabolism and insulin sensitivity. The effect of EDCs on PYY function may also lead to metabolic disorders such as insulin resistance, and this may contribute to weight gain and the development of type 2 diabetes (Heindel and Blumberg 2019).

5. Stomach

The stomach is also involved in the regulation of appetite and energy balance through the production of hormones, including ghrelin. An easy way to remember ghrelin is to think of it as a gremlin. The little gremlin in your stomach causes it to growl sometimes, screaming at you, "Feed me!" Ghrelin is a hormone that is sometimes referred to as the "hunger hormone" because it increases appetite and facilitates the storage of fat. Endocrine-disrupting chemicals (EDCs) can affect the function of the stomach and increase ghrelin levels that lead to weight gain and obesity. They can also boost the effectiveness of ghrelin, which increases the desire to eat. In addition, EDCs can interact with the receptors that ghrelin usually attach to, and in a way, fool the body into thinking that it needs to take in more calories than it should.

Mechanisms of EDC Action on the Stomach and Ghrelin

Stimulation of ghrelin secretion: The stomach releases ghrelin, which can be stimulated by EDCs such as BPA and phthalates. These chemicals can act on the feedback mechanisms that control the secretion of ghrelin, resulting in increased secretion of this hormone. The levels of ghrelin are increased to increase hunger and food intake, leading to weight gain (Engel et al. 2018).

Disruption of ghrelin regulation: EDCs can interfere with the feedback mechanisms that control ghrelin production. Ghrelin levels are also known to rise before meals to increase appetite and then decrease after eating. This means that EDCs can disrupt the normal cycle such that ghrelin levels remain elevated and hunger signals are still present, which can lead to overeating (Melzer et al. 2010).

Impact on gastrointestinal motility: EDCs effects on the gastrointestinal tract may include changes in motility of the stomach. As a result of altering the motility of the gastrointestinal tract, EDCs can interfere with the secretion and clearance of ghrelin and thereby interfere with the regulation of appetite (Sargis 2014).

Effects on Ghrelin and Weight Gain

Increased appetite and food intake: Elevated ghrelin levels due to EDC exposure can lead to increased appetite and food intake. Ghrelin acts on the hypothalamus to stimulate hunger, and higher levels of this hormone can cause individuals to eat more frequently and in larger quantities, contributing to weight gain (Engel et al. 2018).

Enhanced fat storage: Being ghrelin stimulators, EDCs are responsible for increasing not only appetite but also fat storage. Higher levels of ghrelin have been found to increase fat accumulation, especially in the abdominal area. This effect is made even worse by the fact that EDCs can also target other hormonal pathways that are involved in the control of fat metabolism (Melzer et al. 2010).

Development of obesity: Chronic exposure to EDCs and the increased ghrelin levels resulting from this can lead to obesity. The mechanisms of action of overeating and increased fat storage due to increased ghrelin levels may lead to weight gain and increased risk of metabolic comorbidities including type 2 diabetes and cardiovascular disease (Sargis 2014).

6. Liver

The liver is a very important organ in the body that helps in metabolism, detoxification, and energy homeostasis. Endocrine-disrupting chemicals (EDCs) can have adverse effects on the liver and can lead to slow metabolism and weight gain.

Mechanisms of EDC Action on the Liver

Disruption of liver enzymes: EDCs such as bisphenol A (BPA), phthalates, and polychlorinated biphenyls (PCBs) can act on the liver to alter the activity of enzymes that help in detoxification and metabolic functions. These chemicals can block or change the function of cytochrome P450 (CYP) enzymes, which are involved in the metabolism of fat and other nutrients (Gore et al. 2015). CYP enzymes are crucial for metabolizing drugs, hormone regulation, and detoxification from harmful substances like toxins and some cancer-causing agents.

Induction of liver inflammation: EDCs can also lead to inflammation of the liver and produce symptoms of nonalcoholic fatty liver disease (NAFLD). Hepatic inflammation can hinder the liver in its role of processing and storing fats, thus leading to metabolic disturbances and weight gain (Heindel and Vandenberg 2015).

Oxidative stress: EDCs can cause oxidative stress in the liver, which damages hepatocytes and leads to compromised liver function. Oxidative damage can also affect the liver in its ability to regulate glucose and lipid metabolism, and thus leads to obesity and insulin resistance (Sargis et al. 2010).

Effects on Metabolism and Weight Gain

Slowed metabolism: EDCs affect liver enzymes and cause inflammation that can decrease the rate of metabolism. A slow metabolism leads to decreased energy expenditure, and hence weight gain, even with normal calorie intake (Gore et al. 2015).

Fat accumulation: Liver dysfunction may lead to the accumulation of fat in the liver and other organs. NAFLD induced by EDCs can cause the liver to accumulate fats instead of metabolizing them, and thus contributes to weight gain and obesity (Heindel and Vandenberg 2015).

Insulin resistance: EDCs can worsen insulin resistance by affecting the function of the liver. Insulin resistance hampers the ability of cells to uptake glucose from the blood, which leads to increased blood sugar and fat accumulation. This is a metabolic derangement that is closely associated with weight gain and type 2 diabetes (Sargis et al. 2010).

Fatty Liver

PFAs, PFOA, and PFOS—also known as "forever chemicals"—are linked with nonalcoholic fatty liver disease. They are more potent in high-fat diet conditions. Some cause weight gain without increasing food intake. High levels of BPA can lead to abnormal liver function tests and can also deplete the liver of its antioxidant glutathione.

7. Pancreas

Insulin resistance is a metabolic disorder that can lead to the development of type 2 diabetes and is characterized by a diminished response to insulin. When this happens, more insulin is required to maintain the same level of blood glucose, which leads to increased levels of insulin in the blood, a situation that is known to cause weight gain. Interestingly, it has been established that EDCs can act as inducers of insulin resistance. Insulin is very important in decreasing blood glucose, but insulin resistance can cause inflammation and fat storage.

BPAs are not only bad for reproductive health; they can also be detrimental for our metabolism. They affect every end point in the metabolic pathway and are the strongest obesogens. According to animal and human studies, BPA can cause insulin resistance by affecting the fat cells. BPA not only increases the number of fat cells; it can also make fat cells work abnormally. In 2008, Hugo et al. investigated the effects of BPA on hormones that control blood glucose and fat metabolism.

Phthalates are mostly used in plastics and some cosmetics, and have been found to be associated with insulin resistance, which is yet another threat to metabolic health. A 2012 study by Lind et al. reported a relationship between phthalate levels and diabetes in an older adult population.

Some long-lasting, persistent pollutants like PCBs may increase the risk of insulin resistance and type 2 diabetes. According to a 2007 study by Lee et al., these pollutants were linked with insulin resistance in people with no diabetes.

Mechanisms of Action
Pancreatic confusion: Some EDCs may act on the pancreas, the organ that produces insulin, and make the tissues less sensitive to the hormone.

Igniting inflammation: EDCs may cause inflammation in fat tissues. Chronic inflammation is a well-known factor that can lead to insulin resistance.

Cellular sabotage: Imagine EDCs as cellular jamming devices. They might interfere with insulin receptors on cell membranes, hindering insulin's effectiveness in regulating blood sugar.

Scan to learn more about metabolic syndrome and insulin resistance.

All videos are provided courtesy of Alilia Medical Media. Copying and/or downloading of any of the videos or animations to any social media platforms such as YouTube, Facebook, or TikTok is strictly prohibited.

©Alila Medical Media. All medical materials are for information purposes *only* and are *not* intended to be medical advice.

8. Adrenal Glands

The adrenal glands, located on top of the kidneys, are crucial for producing hormones such as cortisol, which regulate stress response, metabolism, and energy balance. Endocrine-disrupting chemicals (EDCs) can significantly impact adrenal function and cortisol production, leading to metabolic disturbances and weight gain.

Mechanisms of EDC Action on the Adrenal Glands
- **Disruption of Cortisol Synthesis**
  - » **EDCs and enzyme inhibition:** EDCs such as bisphenol A (BPA), phthalates, and polychlorinated biphenyls (PCBs) can interfere with enzymes responsible for cortisol synthesis. These chemicals disrupt the hypothalamic-pituitary-adrenal (HPA) axis, which regulates cortisol production. For example, EDCs can inhibit the enzyme 11β-hydroxysteroid dehydrogenase, which converts inactive cortisone to active cortisol (Gore et al. 2015). Therefore, less active cortisol leads to symptoms of fatigue, lightheadedness, and even low blood pressure.
- **Alteration of Adrenal Hormone Receptors**
  - » **Receptor binding and blocking:** EDCs can bind to or block adrenal hormone receptors, affecting cortisol release. Pesticides and industrial chemicals can act as agonists (stimulators) or antagonists (blockers) to glucocorticoid receptors (GR), leading to imbalanced cortisol production. For instance, atrazine, a commonly used herbicide, can modify GR activity, affecting cortisol levels (Diamanti-Kandarakis et al. 2009).
- **Impact on Adrenal Cell Function**
  - » **Cytotoxic effects on adrenal cells:** EDCs can directly damage adrenal cells, impairing their ability to produce cortisol. Chronic exposure to EDCs can lead to adrenal gland hyperplasia (overgrowth), which could lead to increased cortisol production or adrenal atrophy (wasting or shrinking) that can cause decreased cortisol regulation. Studies have shown that BPA exposure can lead to adrenal gland thickening and altered adrenal hormone secretion (Rosenfeld 2017).

Effects on Cortisol and Weight Gain
- **Elevated Cortisol Levels**
  - » **Hypercortisolism:** Chronic EDC exposure can result in elevated cortisol levels (hypercortisolism). High cortisol levels increase appetite, cravings for high-calorie foods, and fat storage, especially in the abdominal region. Elevated cortisol levels are linked to higher body mass index (BMI) and obesity (Newbold et al. 2009).
- **Cortisol and Insulin Resistance**
  - » **Metabolic disruption:** Elevated cortisol levels contribute to insulin resistance, where cells become less responsive to insulin. In turn, insulin resistance impairs glucose metabolism, leading to higher blood sugar levels and increased fat storage. This metabolic imbalance is a significant factor in weight gain and the development of type 2 diabetes (Sargis et al. 2010).
- **Impact on Fat Distribution**
  - » **Central obesity:** Cortisol influences fat distribution, promoting central obesity with increased fat accumulation around the abdomen (a.k.a. belly fat) and around internal organs (a.k.a. visceral fat). Central obesity is associated with higher risks of cardiovascular diseases and metabolic syndrome. Visceral fat is more metabolically active than subcutaneous fat (fat under the skin), meaning it makes hormones and chemicals that contribute to inflammation and increased risk of chronic diseases. EDCs that elevate cortisol levels can exacerbate central obesity and related health issues (Heindel and Vandenberg 2015).
- **Stress and Eating Behaviors**
  - » **Stress-eating cycle:** Chronic stress, worsened by disturbed cortisol regulation, can bring about stress-related eating

behaviors. Elevated cortisol levels increase hunger and cravings for high-fat, sugary foods, contributing to weight gain. This stress-eating cycle is prolonged by ongoing EDC exposure, further increasing obesity risk (Diamanti-Kandarakis et al. 2009).

9. Reproductive Organs: Testosterone and Estrogen

Endocrine-disrupting chemicals (EDCs) can interfere with the endocrine system, leading to imbalances in key hormones such as testosterone and estrogen. It should be noted that men and women make varying amounts of both hormones. Men make more testosterone, whereas women make more estrogen. Hormonal disruptions to either one can have significant effects on both men and women, contributing to weight gain and metabolic disorders.

Mechanisms of EDC Action on Testosterone and Estrogen
- **Mimicking and Blocking Hormones**
  - **Estrogenic activity:** EDCs like bisphenol A (BPA), phthalates, and certain pesticides can mimic estrogen by binding to estrogen receptors. This can lead to an overestimation of estrogen in the body, disrupting the natural hormonal balance (Diamanti-Kandarakis et al. 2009). Excess estrogen, sometimes referred to as "estrogen dominance," can lead to symptoms such as irregular periods, breast tenderness, weight gain, mood swings, and fatigue. It can also be linked with conditions such as endometriosis, fibroids, and certain cancers. In men, high levels of estrogen can cause enlargement of the breasts, infertility, difficulty with erections, decreased sex drive, mood changes, and weight gain.

- » **Antiandrogenic activity:** EDCs can block androgen receptors, reducing the activity of testosterone. Chemicals such as phthalates and PCBs have been shown to interfere with androgen signaling, leading to decreased testosterone levels (Gray et al. 2000). In women, low testosterone levels can cause symptoms including decreased sex drive, fatigue, vaginal dryness with painful intercourse, decreased muscle mass, difficulty reaching an orgasm, weight gain, and mood changes. Similarly, in men, associated symptoms of low testosterone include low sperm count, difficulty with erections, bone loss, insomnia, depression, breast development, and weight gain.
- **Disruption of Hormone Synthesis and Metabolism**
  - » **Inhibition of enzyme activity:** EDCs can inhibit enzymes involved in the making and production of hormones. For example, BPA can inhibit aromatase, an enzyme that converts testosterone to estrogen, disrupting the balance of these hormones (Diamanti-Kandarakis et al. 2009).
  - » **Alteration of hormone transport:** EDCs can affect the proteins that carry hormones safely throughout the bloodstream, altering their accessibility to tissues and activity at their receptors. This can lead to hormonal imbalances and metabolic disturbances (Zoeller et al. 2012).

Effects on Testosterone, Estrogen, and Weight Gain
- **Effects in Men**
  - » **Decreased testosterone levels:** Lower testosterone levels due to EDC exposure can lead to increased fat deposition and reduced muscle mass. Since muscle tissue burns more calories at rest than fat tissue, a decline in muscle mass leads to a slower metabolism. This makes it easier to store

excess calories as fat. Testosterone plays a crucial role in regulating body composition by promoting muscle growth and fat metabolism. Reduced testosterone levels can impair these processes, leading to weight gain and increased risk of obesity (Sharpe 2010).

» **Insulin resistance and metabolic syndrome:** Low testosterone levels are associated with insulin resistance, a condition where the body's cells become less responsive to insulin. This is due to increased visceral fat accumulation, which is more resistant to insulin action; and due to decreased muscle mass, this makes the body less sensitive to insulin. This can lead to decreased uptake of glucose into the cells for energy, elevated blood sugar levels, increased conversion of sugar into fat, increased fat storage, and metabolic syndrome—a cluster of conditions that increase the risk of heart disease and diabetes (Vandenberg et al. 2012).

- **Effects in Women**
    » **Increased estrogen levels:** Elevated estrogen levels due to EDCs can lead to increased fat storage, particularly in the hips and thighs. Estrogen plays a role in regulating fat distribution, and higher levels can promote fat accumulation in specific areas (Newbold et al. 2009). When high estrogen levels influence glucose metabolism and insulin sensitivity leading to insulin resistance, then the excess glucose is stored as fat, especially around the belly.
    » **Disruption of hormonal balance:** EDCs can disrupt the balance between estrogen and other hormones such as progesterone and testosterone. This imbalance can lead to weight gain, insulin resistance, and other metabolic disorders. For example, elevated estrogen levels

can interfere with thyroid function, leading to reduced metabolism and weight gain (Diamanti-Kandarakis et al. 2009). Excess estrogen can increase the protein that binds to thyroid hormones called thyroxine-binding globulin (TBG). Increased amounts of this protein reduce the amount of free and active thyroid hormones available to cells to use. This can potentially lead to hypothyroidism (underactive thyroid) and decreased metabolism.

- **Common Effects on Both Genders**
  - » **Enhanced adipogenesis:** EDCs can stimulate the maturation of precursor cells into adipocytes, or fat cells, which store energy. This process is controlled by hormones like testosterone and estrogen, and their perturbation can boost adipogenesis and thus obesity (Heindel and Vandenberg 2015).
  - » **Leptin and ghrelin imbalance:** EDCs can interfere with the production of leptin and ghrelin, the hormones that control the feelings of fullness and hunger, respectively. Disturbance of these hormones may result in increased hunger, overeating, and weight gain. Estrogenic EDCs can induce leptin resistance, meaning that the brain no longer recognizes the stomach as being full (Gore et al. 2015).

Xenoestrogens: Their Development from EDCs and Their Role in Weight Gain

Xenoestrogens ("foreign estrogens") are a subcategory of endocrine-disrupting chemicals (EDCs) that mimic the action of natural estrogens in the body. Remember those imposters we spoke about in chapter two? They impersonate as if they were truly estrogen. They are synthetic or natural chemical compounds that have structures closely resembling estrogen. They can then bind to estrogen receptors, causing similar or even more potent effects than estrogens made by the body. Xenoestrogens are found in various sources, including pesticides, industrial chemicals, plastics, and personal care products. Their ability to interfere with the endocrine system can lead to significant health issues, including weight gain and obesity.

Development of Xenoestrogens from EDCs
1. **Sources of Xenoestrogens**
   » **Industrial chemicals:** Many industrial chemicals, such as bisphenol A (BPA), phthalates, and polychlorinated biphenyls (PCBs), act as xenoestrogens. BPA, for instance, is widely used in the production of polycarbonate plastics and epoxy resins, found in items like water bottles and food can linings (Rochester 2013).
   » **Pesticides:** Certain pesticides, including DDT and its metabolites, as well as some herbicides, exhibit xenoestrogenic activity. These chemicals can persist in the environment and magnify contamination in the food chain, leading to widespread human exposure (Diamanti-Kandarakis et al. 2009).
   » **Personal care products:** Parabens and certain synthetic fragrances used in cosmetics and personal care products also act as xenoestrogens. These chemicals are absorbed through the skin and can accumulate in body tissues (Darbre and Harvey 2008).
2. **Mechanisms of Action**
   » **Estrogen receptor binding:** Xenoestrogens can bind to estrogen receptors (ERs) on cells, particularly $ER\alpha$ (alpha) and $ER\beta$ (beta), mimicking the effects of natural estrogens. This can lead to altered gene expression and can disrupt the normal hormonal balance in the body (Safe 2004).

Estrogen receptors are found in various tissues throughout the body, including in the reproductive organs, pituitary gland, adrenal gland, heart, blood vessels, brain, bones, liver, and skin. They are also present in the nucleus of cells where they bind to estrogen and regulate gene expression.

» **Estrogenic potency:** While some xenoestrogens are weaker than natural estrogens, others can be more potent, leading to exaggerated estrogenic effects. The cumulative exposure to multiple xenoestrogens, even in low doses, can result in significant hormonal disruption (Vandenberg et al. 2012). They can be more potent than natural estrogen because they can bind to the estrogen receptor with higher affinity, and may even lead to stronger effects. Bisphenol A (BPA), ethinyl estradiol (EE2), diethylstilbestrol (DES), and alkylphenols are examples of xenoestrogens with high affinities.

Xenoestrogens and Weight Gain
1. **Promotion of Adipogenesis**
   » Xenoestrogens can promote the differentiation of preadipocytes (precursor cells) into adipocytes (fat cells). This process, known as adipogenesis, leads to an increase in the number of fat cells and overall fat mass. Xenoestrogens such as BPA have been shown to enhance the expression of genes involved in adipogenesis, leading to increased fat storage (Grün and Blumberg 2009).
2. **Disruption of Metabolic Hormones**
   » Xenoestrogens can interfere with the balance of metabolic hormones, including insulin, leptin, and adiponectin. For example, BPA has been shown to reduce levels of adiponectin, a hormone that enhances insulin sensitivity

and fat metabolism. Lower adiponectin levels are associated with increased fat accumulation and a higher risk of obesity (Rochester 2013).

3. **Estrogenic Effects on Fat Distribution**
   » Estrogen plays a key role in regulating fat distribution, particularly in women. Xenoestrogens can mimic estrogen's effects on fat distribution, leading to increased fat storage in areas such as the hips, thighs, and abdomen. This type of fat distribution is often more resistant to weight loss and is associated with a higher risk of metabolic disorders (Newbold et al. 2009).

4. **Insulin Resistance and Obesity**
   » Chronic exposure to xenoestrogens can contribute to the development of insulin resistance, a condition where the body's cells become less responsive to insulin. Insulin resistance leads to elevated blood glucose levels and increased fat storage, further promoting weight gain and obesity. This effect is particularly concerning given the widespread exposure to xenoestrogens in the environment (Grün and Blumberg 2009).

10. Fat Cells as an Endocrine Organ

For many years, fat cells (adipocytes) were primarily regarded as passive storage units for excess energy in the form of triglycerides. However, research over the past few decades has transformed our understanding, revealing that adipose tissue is not merely a fat reservoir but an active endocrine organ that plays a key role in regulating various physiological processes. With this discovery, we can designate fat cells as an endocrine organ. Adipocytes secrete a variety of hormones and cytokines—collectively known as adipokines—that influence metabolism, inflammation, appetite, insulin sensitivity, and energy homeostasis. The key hormones secreted by fat cells are leptin and adiponectin.

Impact on Fat Cells (Adipocytes)
EDCs have the ability to influence the differentiation of preadipocytes into mature adipocytes, or fat cells. This process, known as adipogenesis, can increase the body's overall fat mass. Some EDCs act as agonists for receptors that trigger the expression of genes involved in fat storage, causing an increase in the number and size of fat cells.

Adipogenesis
Obesogens can stimulate the differentiation of stem cells into fat cells, thereby increasing the body's capacity to store fat. EDCs are lipophilic, meaning that they are strongly attracted to fat. Therefore, they are stored and accumulate in the fatty tissues in the liver, fat, brain, and skin.

Leptin: The Satiety Hormone and Its Role in Weight Regulation

What Is Leptin?
Leptin is a hormone predominantly produced by adipocytes (fat cells), and it plays a crucial role in regulating energy balance by inhibiting hunger. It acts on receptors in the hypothalamus in the brain, where it helps to regulate appetite and body weight. Leptin is often referred to as the "satiety hormone" or "starvation hormone" because it signals the brain that the body has enough energy stored in fat cells, helping to prevent overeating.

How Leptin Affects Weight
1. **Regulation of Appetite**
    » Leptin's primary role is to regulate appetite. It is released by fat cells in response to the amount of fat stored in the body. When fat stores increase, leptin levels rise, signaling

the brain to reduce the urge to eat and increase energy expenditure. Conversely, when fat stores decrease, leptin levels fall, triggering hunger and a reduction in energy expenditure (Zhang et al. 1994). Have you ever heard the phrase "feast or famine"? Well, during the feast period, fat cells mobilize to store the excess fat, which triggers leptin to tell the body to boost energy outflow to use fat as a source for energy. However, during the famine period, when fat stores are lower than normal, leptin increases appetite to correct the imbalance. The key is to get that sweet spot that satisfies leptin levels.

2. **Energy Expenditure**
   » Leptin not only reduces food intake but also influences energy consumption. It acts on the hypothalamus to increase metabolic rate and energy output. This dual role helps maintain energy homeostasis and body weight within a normal range (Ahima and Flier 2000).

3. **Leptin Resistance**
   » In some cases, particularly in obese individuals, the body can develop leptin resistance. This means that, despite high levels of leptin, the brain does not respond adequately to the hormone's signals, leading to continued overeating and reduced energy expenditure. Leptin resistance is a significant factor in the development and persistence of obesity (Friedman 2019). Although the exact cause is not fully understood, we do see that several factors such as chronic inflammation, lack of physical activity, and a diet high in processed foods, sugar, and unhealthy fats can all contribute to leptin resistance.

How EDCs Affect Leptin and Contribute to Weight Gain

1. **Disruption of Leptin Production**
   » Endocrine-disrupting chemicals (EDCs) such as bisphenol A (BPA), phthalates, and organotin can disrupt leptin production in adipose tissue. Studies have shown that exposure to these chemicals can lead to altered leptin levels, either increasing or decreasing its production in ways that disrupt normal metabolic regulation (Grün and Blumberg 2009).

2. **Leptin Resistance and EDCs**
   » EDCs have been implicated in the development of leptin resistance. For example, BPA exposure has been linked to increased levels of leptin and the development of leptin resistance, contributing to obesity. This resistance means that, even though leptin is present at high levels, its ability to regulate appetite and energy expenditure is impaired (Vom Saal and Myers 2008).

3. **Impact on Energy Balance**
   » EDCs are known to interfere with leptin signaling, which results in an imbalance between energy intake and expenditure. This disruption may enhance appetite, reduce energy expenditure, and lead to weight gain. For example, in obese patients, EDCs like organotin have been found to activate peroxisome proliferator-activated receptors (PPARs), which regulate fat cell differentiation and leptin production and thereby contribute to weight gain and obesity (Janesick and Blumberg 2016).

4. **Alteration of Hypothalamic Function**
   » EDCs can also affect the hypothalamus, the region of the brain where leptin exerts its effects. By disrupting hypothalamic function, EDCs can impair leptin signaling

pathways, leading to altered appetite regulation and increased food intake. This effect is particularly concerning as it directly interferes with the body's natural ability to maintain energy balance (Heindel and Blumberg 2019).

Review of Adiponectin and Its Role in Weight Regulation

What Is Adiponectin?

Adiponectin is a protein hormone produced and secreted primarily by adipocytes (fat cells). It plays a crucial role in regulating glucose levels, fatty acid breakdown, and overall energy metabolism. Unlike other adipokines, adiponectin is unique because its levels are inversely related to body fat percentage; higher levels of adiponectin are generally associated with lower levels of body fat and a reduced risk of obesity-related conditions such as type 2 diabetes and cardiovascular disease.

How Adiponectin Affects Weight

1. **Insulin Sensitivity**
    » Adiponectin enhances the body's sensitivity to insulin, making it easier for cells to take up glucose from the blood. This action helps maintain normal blood sugar levels and prevents the excessive fat accumulation that often accompanies insulin resistance (Kadowaki et al. 2006).
2. **Fatty Acid Oxidation**
    » Adiponectin promotes the oxidation of fatty acids, especially in skeletal muscles and the liver. This process involves breaking down stored fat for energy, which can help reduce overall fat mass and support weight management (Fruebis et al. 2001).

3. **Anti-Inflammatory Effects**
   » Adiponectin has anti-inflammatory properties that help mitigate the chronic inflammation commonly associated with obesity and metabolic syndrome. Lower inflammation levels contribute to better metabolic health and reduce the risk of weight gain and related disorders (Ouchi et al. 2011).
4. **Regulation of Appetite and Energy Expenditure**
   » Although adiponectin is primarily involved in metabolic regulation, it also influences appetite and energy expenditure indirectly through its effects on other hormones like leptin and insulin. This contributes to a more balanced energy intake and expenditure, promoting healthy weight maintenance (Kadowaki et al. 2006).

How EDCs Affect Adiponectin Levels and Contribute to Weight Gain

1. **Reduction in Adiponectin Levels**
   » Exposure to endocrine-disrupting chemicals (EDCs) like bisphenol A (BPA) and phthalates have been shown to reduce adiponectin levels in the body. Lower adiponectin levels are linked to decreased insulin sensitivity, increased fat storage, and a higher risk of developing obesity (Rochester 2013).
2. **Increased Insulin Resistance**
   » By lowering adiponectin levels, EDCs can contribute to the development of insulin resistance. When insulin resistance occurs, the body's ability to effectively regulate blood sugar is impaired, leading to increased glucose levels and fat storage, particularly in the abdominal region (Heindel and Vandenberg 2015).

3. **Promotion of Inflammation**
   » EDCs can exacerbate inflammation in adipose tissue by disrupting the balance of adipokines, including adiponectin. Chronic inflammation is closely associated with obesity and metabolic syndrome, and the reduction of adiponectin by EDCs can aggravate this condition, making weight gain more likely (Grün and Blumberg 2009).
4. **Impact on Fat Storage and Metabolism**
   » The reduction in adiponectin levels caused by EDCs disrupts the normal process of fatty acid oxidation, leading to increased fat accumulation. This contributes to obesity and its associated metabolic disorders, such as type 2 diabetes and cardiovascular disease (Rochester 2013).

PPAR Gamma Receptors: The Master Regulators of Fat Storage

What Is PPAR Gamma?

Peroxisome proliferator-activated receptor gamma (PPARγ) is a nuclear receptor that plays a critical role in the regulation of the storage of fat and glucose metabolism. PPARγ is primarily expressed in adipose tissue, but it is also found in the liver, muscle, and other tissues. It is often referred to as the "master regulator" of adipogenesis because of its crucial role in the differentiation of preadipocytes into mature adipocytes (fat cells) and in the regulation of lipid metabolism. EDCs can act as agonists or antagonists for PPARγ, thereby influencing the storage of fat and the body's sensitivity to insulin. Some EDCs are known to activate PPARγ, promoting the differentiation of preadipocytes into mature adipocytes and leading to increased fat storage.

By acting on these four key mechanisms, EDCs orchestrate a multifaceted disruption of metabolic processes. This includes the proliferation and enlargement of fat cells, dysregulation of hunger and satiety hormones, and manipulation of receptors critical for fat storage and insulin sensitivity. Each of these mechanisms can contribute to weight gain and obesity.

Role of PPAR Gamma in Obesity
1. **Adipogenesis**
   - » **Fat cell formation:** PPARγ is essential for the formation of fat cells. When activated, PPARγ promotes the expression of genes involved in adipogenesis, leading to the conversion of preadipocytes into mature adipocytes. This process increases the body's capacity to store fat (Tontonoz and Spiegelman 2008).
   - » **Lipid storage:** PPARγ also enhances the storage of lipids within adipocytes by regulating the expression of genes involved in lipid uptake and storage. This helps to sequester excess fatty acids and triglycerides in adipose tissue, thereby preventing lipotoxicity in other tissues (Ahmadian et al. 2013).
2. **Insulin Sensitivity**
   - » **Glucose metabolism:** PPARγ plays a key role in enhancing insulin sensitivity. It regulates the expression of genes involved in glucose uptake and metabolism, particularly in adipose tissue and skeletal muscle. This action helps to lower blood glucose levels and improve overall metabolic health (Lehrke and Lazar 2005).
   - » **Thiazolidinediones:** Medications like thiazolidinediones (TZDs), used to treat type 2 diabetes, work by activating PPARγ. These drugs improve insulin sensitivity and reduce blood sugar levels by promoting the storage of excess glucose as fat in adipose tissue (Lehrke and Lazar 2005).

3. **Obesity**
   » **Increased fat storage:** While PPARγ activation improves insulin sensitivity, it also promotes fat storage, which can lead to weight gain and obesity when not properly regulated. In individuals with a predisposition to obesity, excessive activation of PPARγ can result in an increase in the size and number of adipocytes, leading to excessive fat accumulation (Ahmadian et al. 2013).
   » **Adipose tissue expansion:** In obesity, PPARγ contributes to the expansion of adipose tissue by promoting both hyperplasia (increase in fat cell number) and hypertrophy (increase in fat cell size). This expansion can lead to the development of obesity-related complications, such as insulin resistance, type 2 diabetes, and cardiovascular disease (Tontonoz and Spiegelman 2008).

How EDCs Affect PPAR Gamma and Lead to Weight Gain
1. **Activation of PPAR Gamma by EDCs**
   » **Obesogens:** EDCs, particularly a class of chemicals known as obesogens, can activate PPARγ, mimicking the effects of natural ligands and leading to increased fat storage. Chemicals like tributyltin (TBT) and bisphenol A (BPA) are known to bind to PPARγ and enhance adipogenesis, contributing to weight gain and obesity (Grün and Blumberg 2009).
   » **Enhanced adipogenesis:** EDCs that activate PPARγ promote the differentiation of preadipocytes into mature adipocytes, increasing the body's capacity to store fat. This effect is particularly concerning because it can occur even with low-dose exposure to these chemicals,

leading to gradual weight gain over time (Janesick and Blumberg 2011).

2. **Disruption of Metabolic Homeostasis**
   » **Insulin resistance:** While PPARγ activation generally improves insulin sensitivity, the chronic activation of PPARγ by EDCs can disrupt metabolic homeostasis, leading to insulin resistance. This paradoxical effect occurs because the excessive storage of fat can eventually impair the ability of insulin to effectively regulate blood glucose levels, contributing to the development of type 2 diabetes (Heindel and Blumberg 2019).
   » **Chronic inflammation:** EDCs can also induce inflammation in adipose tissue by altering the expression of pro-inflammatory cytokines through PPARγ-dependent and independent pathways. Chronic inflammation is a hallmark of obesity and contributes to the development of metabolic syndrome and related diseases (Grün and Blumberg 2009).
3. **Impact on Fat Distribution**
   » **Visceral fat accumulation:** EDC-induced activation of PPARγ can lead to an increase in visceral fat, the type of fat stored around internal organs. Visceral fat is particularly dangerous because it is metabolically active and is associated with a higher risk of cardiovascular diseases, insulin resistance, and other obesity-related conditions (Janesick and Blumberg 2011).
   » **Altered fat distribution:** The impact of EDCs on PPARγ can lead to an altered pattern of fat distribution, with increased deposition of fat in areas such as the abdomen, which is linked to higher morbidity and mortality rates (Heindel and Blumberg 2019).

Final Notes

Chronic Low-Dose Exposure
Traditionally, toxicological studies operate on the principle that "the dose makes the poison." However, obesogens appear to defy this principle; even low-dose, chronic exposure can have a significant impact on body weight and metabolic health.

The timing of exposure to EDCs can be just as important as the dose. Critical windows of vulnerability, such as prenatal and early postnatal periods, can have a lasting impact on metabolic health.

High-Risk Populations
Infants and children: Exposure early in life can have lifelong consequences, affecting metabolism and risk of obesity in adulthood.
Pregnant women: Exposure during pregnancy can have multigenerational impacts, affecting not just the child but potentially even the grandchild.

Conclusion
So did all of this information about EDCs and weight just make your head hurt? Feeling overwhelmed about what you have just learned? Trust me when I say that I, too, shared the same feelings. I was stunned by the numerous ways EDCs are making us fat. I share this to emphasize that your efforts are not in vain, and it's not your fault. As you can now appreciate, external forces are working against our efforts to maintain heathy weights and waistlines. The concept of EDCs as obesogens expands the current understanding of the factors that lead to the obesity epidemic. Lifestyle factors such as diet and exercise are clearly significant, but the impact of EDCs cannot be overlooked. These detailed mechanisms highlight the need to view weight management as more complex than the simplistic notion of

"calories in and calories out." This highlights the importance of a multifactorial approach to the rising obesity and metabolic syndrome rates. The unfortunate reality is that our "chemical footprint" may be as bad as our carbon footprint. In the fight against obesity, knowing how to combat EDCs gives us one more weapon to regain our health and quality of life. Fear not, my friend! The good news is that there are many ways to counteract these disturbances, which will be discussed in great detail in chapter ten. However, in the next chapter, let us first review how EDCs can affect our energy levels linked with chronic fatigue. This, too, can impact our metabolic health and the hormonal balance that regulates these physiological processes.

CHAPTER EIGHT:

How EDCs Are Making Us Tired: The Role of EDCs in Fatigue and Energy Levels

Our energy is being called for in countless ways in a world that needs it now more than ever. But then there are the ever-present EDCs that cast a shadow on our attempts to maintain consistent, vibrant energy levels. From their impact on our energy during the day to our quality of sleep at night, these chemicals work their way through our energy tapestry in stealth fashion to undo what we are trying to do to stay lively and alert.

1. EDCs: The Invisible Energy Thieves

Anchored in our routine lives, EDCs secretly dismantle our energy reserves, disrupting our biological rhythms and hormonal balance. Their prevalent influence is particularly ominous due to their subtle, often unnoticed effects on our overall vitality.

EDCs, by their very nature, disrupt the endocrine system, affecting hormonal secretion and action that is vital for regulating energy levels. Furthermore, by interfering with metabolic hormones, EDCs can modify our energy expenditure, leading to feelings of fatigue and lethargy.

2. Infiltrating Our Sleep: The Unseen Assault on Rest

Quality sleep is paramount for rejuvenation, mental clarity, and overall health. EDCs, however, silently intrude upon our sleep, potentially disrupting the critical restorative processes that occur overnight.

EDCs may impair production of melatonin, a hormone pivotal for sleep regulation, impacting our sleep-wake cycle. EDC-induced sleep disturbances such as restlessness at night can culminate in chronic fatigue, hampering cognitive functions and emotional well-being.

3. EDCs and Adrenal Function

Exploring deeper, the sneaky nature of EDCs extends to their impact on our adrenal glands, and particularly our "stress hormone," cortisol.

Constant EDC exposure may stress the adrenal glands, leading to imbalances in cortisol production. Cortisol is important for converting food into energy; so, when levels are low, the body struggles to access and use energy effectively. With altered cortisol levels, our stress response, metabolism, blood sugar regulation, and energy allocation are thrown into disarray, potentially manifesting as persistent fatigue. In addition, low cortisol levels can disrupt the sleep-wake cycle, resulting in poor sleep quality and daytime fatigue. It should be noted that the term "adrenal fatigue" is not a recognized medical condition. However, some people can experience similar symptoms to adrenal insufficiency such as irritability, fatigue, brain fog, and difficulty coping with stress.

4. EDCs and Thyroid Dysfunction

The thyroid gland plays a pivotal role in regulating metabolism, energy production, and overall cellular function. Endocrine-disrupting chemicals (EDCs) have been shown to interfere with thyroid function, leading to various health issues, including fatigue. These chemicals can disrupt the synthesis, release, and activity of thyroid hormones, which are crucial for maintaining metabolic homeostasis.

Exposure to EDCs, such as polychlorinated biphenyls (PCBs), bisphenol A (BPA), and certain pesticides, has been linked to alterations in thyroid hormone levels. These disruptions can manifest as hypothyroidism (underactive thyroid) or hyperthyroidism (overactive thyroid), both of which can significantly impact energy levels and overall well-being.

Unraveling the Mechanisms Behind EDC-Induced Thyroid Dysfunction and Fatigue

- **Interference with thyroid hormone synthesis:** EDCs can inhibit the production of thyroid hormones by disrupting the enzymes involved in hormone synthesis. For example, PCBs and dioxins have been shown to reduce the activity of thyroid peroxidase, an enzyme critical for the production of thyroid hormones (Ruhlen et al. 2011). This reduction can lead to lower levels of circulating thyroid hormones, resulting in hypothyroidism.
- **Disruption of hormone transport and metabolism:** EDCs can interfere with the transport and metabolism of thyroid hormones. Some chemicals, like BPA, can bind to thyroid hormone transport proteins, reducing the availability of free hormones for cellular uptake (Meeker et al. 2011). Additionally, EDCs can affect the conversion of the less-active thyroxine (T4) to the more-active triiodothyronine (T3), further impairing thyroid function.
- **Thyroid hormone receptor antagonism:** Certain EDCs can act as antagonists to thyroid hormone receptors, preventing

the proper binding of thyroid hormones and impairing their cellular actions. This antagonism can disrupt the normal signaling pathways regulated by thyroid hormones, leading to metabolic dysregulation and fatigue (Boas et al. 2012).

- **Oxidative stress and inflammation:** EDCs can induce oxidative stress and inflammation, which can further impair thyroid function. Oxidative damage to thyroid cells can disrupt hormone production, while chronic inflammation can alter the structure and function of the thyroid gland, contributing to thyroid disorders and fatigue (Zheng et al. 2020).

The impact of EDCs on thyroid function and their subsequent contribution to fatigue underscores the importance of understanding the broader implications of chemical exposure on human health. By elucidating the mechanisms through which EDCs disrupt thyroid function, we can develop more effective strategies to protect public health. This involves raising awareness, advocating for stricter regulations, and making informed choices to reduce exposure to EDCs. Through these collective efforts, we can pave the way for a healthier future, mitigating the impact of these pervasive environmental contaminants on our energy levels and overall well-being.

5. EDCs and Mitochondrial Dysfunction: Impact on ATP Production and Fatigue

The mitochondria, often referred to as the "powerhouses of cells," are critical for generating adenosine triphosphate (ATP), the primary energy currency of cells. Efficient mitochondrial function is essential for maintaining energy levels and overall cellular health. Emerging research suggests that endocrine-disrupting chemicals (EDCs) can impair mitochondrial function, leading to decreased ATP production and contributing to chronic fatigue.

EDCs can affect mitochondrial function through various mechanisms, including oxidative stress, disruption of mitochondrial DNA, and interference with the electron transport chain. This disruption can lead to impaired energy production, which manifests as fatigue and decreased physical and mental performance.

Unraveling the Mechanisms Behind EDC-Induced Mitochondrial Dysfunction and Fatigue

Understanding the specific ways in which EDCs impact mitochondrial function requires a closer look at the underlying biological mechanisms. Let's imagine your body is filled with thousands of tiny battery factories called mitochondria. Each mitochondrion takes in raw materials like oxygen and nutrients and uses them to charge up batteries (called ATP) which power everything your body does—walking, thinking, digesting, healing, and even blinking. When these battery factories work well, your body runs like a well-charged machine, like the Energizer bunny. This helps you feel alert and energetic. But then come the EDCs (endocrine-disrupting chemicals) like thieves in the night armed with wrenches and wires. They sneak into the factory through Trojan horses (like plastic containers and personal care products, pesticide-covered foods, medications, and pollutants). Once inside, they start sabotaging the battery production line. They jam the conveyor belts by interfering with enzymes and hormones like insulin and thyroid hormone that help mitochondria produce energy. They then cause electrical fires that create oxidative stress, damaging the factory's control panels (mitochondrial DNA). To make matters worse, some EDCs even shut down the factory and keep your body from producing ATP entirely. So when your batteries don't fully charge, you wake up feeling like you're already running on empty. Much like your phone when the battery has been drained, your body has to switch to low-power mode, which leads to brain fog, muscle weakness, and decreased concentration. Your body then desperately asks for energy, but the battery factories are not functioning. So let's dig deeper into the science behind how this happens.

- **Oxidative stress:** EDCs can increase the production of reactive oxygen species (ROS) within mitochondria, leading to oxidative stress. ROS are highly reactive molecules that can damage cellular components, including lipids, proteins, and DNA. Oxidative stress disrupts mitochondrial function, impairing the cell's ability to efficiently produce ATP. Studies have shown that EDCs such as BPA and phthalates can elevate ROS levels, leading to oxidative damage and mitochondrial dysfunction (Kloas et al. 2009).
- **Mitochondrial DNA damage:** Mitochondria contain their own DNA, which is critical for encoding proteins involved in the electron transport chain (ETC). EDCs can cause direct damage to mitochondrial DNA (mtDNA), compromising the integrity and functionality of mitochondria. This damage can impair the synthesis of essential mitochondrial proteins, leading to reduced ATP production. Research has indicated that exposure to certain EDCs, such as dioxins and PCBs, can cause mtDNA mutations and impair mitochondrial gene expression (Shen et al. 2014).
- **Disruption of the electron transport chain:** The ETC is essential for oxidative phosphorylation, the process by which ATP is produced. EDCs can interfere with the components of the ETC, reducing the efficiency of ATP synthesis. For instance, studies have found that EDCs such as triclosan can inhibit the activity of ETC complexes, leading to decreased mitochondrial respiration and ATP production (Ajao et al. 2015).

- **Impaired mitochondrial biogenesis:** Mitochondrial biogenesis, the process of forming new mitochondria, is crucial for maintaining a healthy population of these organelles. Some EDCs can interfere with the regulatory pathways involved in mitochondrial biogenesis. For example, studies have shown that EDCs like BPA can inhibit the expression of genes involved in mitochondrial biogenesis, leading to a decrease in mitochondrial number and functionality (Fujimoto et al. 2013). Impaired biogenesis then leads to decreased ATP production and increased fatigue.
- **Epigenetic modifications:** EDCs can induce epigenetic changes that affect mitochondrial function. Epigenetic modifications, such as DNA methylation and histone acetylation, can alter gene expression without changing the DNA sequence. These modifications can impact genes involved in mitochondrial function and energy metabolism, leading to long-term effects on cellular energy production. Research has demonstrated that prenatal exposure to EDCs can result in epigenetic alterations that persist into adulthood, affecting mitochondrial function and contributing to fatigue (Rüegg et al. 2017). The growing body of evidence suggests that EDC-induced mitochondrial dysfunction plays a significant role in the development of chronic fatigue. By impairing the cellular machinery responsible for energy production, EDCs can lead to persistent energy deficits and contribute to the overall burden of fatigue-related disorders.

6. EDCs and the Gut Microbiome

The gut microbiome, a complex ecosystem of trillions of microorganisms, plays a vital role in regulating various aspects of our health, including sleep quality and energy levels. Endocrine-disrupting chemicals (EDCs), with their strong presence in our environment, do not spare this delicate internal ecosystem, leading to significant implications for our overall well-being.

Gut Health and Sleep
The gut microbiome influences sleep by producing neurotransmitters such as serotonin, which are essential in regulating mood and sleep cycles. It also plays a role in the regulation of circadian rhythms, the body's internal clock that dictates sleep-wake patterns. An optimal gut microbiome is therefore essential for maintaining healthy sleep patterns.

When EDCs are absorbed into our system, they can alter the balance and workings of our gut microbiome. This can change the production of neurotransmitters and, in turn, affect sleep quality. EDCs like bisphenol A (BPA) and phthalates have been found to change the composition of the gut microbiota, which may result in dysbiosis that can adversely affect the function of the gut and the body in general (Heindel et al. 2017). It has been seen that poor sleep can decrease the diversity of the gut bacteria, which affects the production of sleep-regulating neurotransmitters (Reynolds et al. 2017).

Sleep Apnea, EDCs, and the Gut Microbiome
Sleep apnea, characterized by intermittent pauses in breathing during sleep, significantly impacts sleep quality and energy levels. Emerging research suggests that both the gut microbiome and EDCs might play a role in this condition.

There is evidence to suggest a link between gut microbiome composition and sleep apnea. Changes in microbial populations can influence systemic inflammation and obesity, both of which are risk factors for sleep apnea (Jumpertz et al. 2011). Inflammation can cause airway obstruction, while obesity can lead to the physical narrowing of airways, both contributing to the occurrence of sleep apnea.

EDCs can alter the gut microbiome, promoting conditions such as weight gain (discussed in chapter five), which is a significant risk factor for sleep apnea. By creating an unhealthy gut and promoting metabolic disorders, EDCs can indirectly contribute to the development or exacerbation of sleep apnea, further hindering restful sleep. Studies have shown that exposure to certain EDCs is associated with increased body weight and altered metabolic function, potentially leading to or worsening sleep apnea (Janesick and Blumberg 2016).

The complex relationship between the gut microbiome, sleep, and EDCs highlights the need for a holistic approach to health. Addressing the impact of EDCs on the gut microbiome, and how to reduce their effects, can help improve sleep quality and overall well-being. Continued research is essential to fully understand these interactions and develop strategies to minimize the adverse health impacts of EDC exposure.

Conclusion

It is important to know the common sources of EDCs in order to realize how almost every activity and decision one makes may contribute to the loop of gut irritation, poor sleep, and fatigue. Knowing about EDCs and their subtle ways of draining one's energy is a good starting point. It is important to understand how they affect the gut and, in turn, sleep and energy. The remaining chapters will reveal the ways in which one can protect the gut, and thus protect sleep and energy in the context of an environment that is rich in EDCs.

CHAPTER NINE:

Impacts of EDCs on Children and Adolescents

Endocrine-disrupting chemicals (EDCs) pose a significant risk to public health, particularly to the most vulnerable populations: children and adolescents. These chemicals, which can interfere with the normal functioning of the endocrine system, have profound implications during the critical periods of growth and development that occur from infancy through adolescence. This chapter delves into the specific impacts of EDC exposure on these young populations, exploring the mechanisms of action, the health outcomes associated with exposure, and strategies for mitigation.

Understanding the Risk

Children and adolescents are particularly susceptible to the effects of EDCs due to their developing bodies and organs. The endocrine system, which is responsible for hormone regulation and signaling throughout the body, plays a crucial role in growth, development, metabolism, and reproduction. Interference by EDCs during these fundamental times of development can lead to lasting health effects.

Mechanisms of EDC Action in Children and Adolescents
1. **Hormonal imitation and blockade:** EDCs can mimic natural hormones in the body, most notably estrogen and androgen, leading to overstimulation of hormone receptors. Alternatively, they can block the normal action of hormones, leading to disruptions in the body's hormonal balance.
2. **Enzyme alteration:** Some EDCs can alter the synthesis and metabolism of natural hormones, affecting the levels of hormones available for the body's use.
3. **Receptor expression changes:** Exposure to EDCs can also lead to changes in the number of hormone receptors, affecting the sensitivity of tissues to hormonal signals.

Health Outcomes Associated with EDC Exposure
1. **Neurodevelopmental effects:** Exposure to EDCs, such as PCBs and PBDEs, during pregnancy and early childhood has been linked to learning deficits, impaired brain development, reduced IQ, and behavioral problems, including ADHD.
2. **Growth and metabolism:** EDCs like phthalates and BPA have been associated with obesity and metabolic disorders in children. These chemicals can disrupt normal metabolic processes, leading to increased fat storage, obesity, diabetes, and insulin resistance.
3. **Reproductive health:** Early exposure to certain EDCs can affect the development of the reproductive system, leading to premature puberty, fertility issues, and other reproductive health problems later in life.
4. **Immune system disruption:** EDCs can also impact the developing immune system, increasing the risk of infections, asthma, and autoimmune diseases.

5. **Cancer risk:** Some studies have linked EDC exposure to an increased risk of certain cancers later in life.

Strategies for Mitigation and Protection

1. **Reducing exposure:** Limiting the use of plastic containers for food and drinks to reduce BPA, choosing organic and pesticide-free foods, and using natural personal care products to reduce exposure to phthalates can significantly reduce overall EDC exposure.
2. **Advocacy and education:** Advocating for policies that limit the use of harmful chemicals and educating communities about the risks of EDCs are crucial steps in protecting public health.
3. **Research and monitoring:** Ongoing research is essential to better understand the full impact of EDC exposure on children and adolescents and to develop effective interventions.

Conclusion

The impact of EDCs on children and adolescents underscores the need for concerted efforts to reduce exposure and protect these vulnerable populations. By understanding the mechanisms through which EDCs exert their effects and the potential health outcomes, parents, healthcare providers, and policymakers can take actionable steps to mitigate these risks. As research continues to shed light on the pervasive threat posed by EDCs, proactive measures and public health policies will be vital in safeguarding the health and development of future generations.

PART TWO:

This Is War! Strategies for Battling EDCs and Reclaiming Health

In chapters two through nine, we have reviewed in detail how EDCs are making us sick, fat, and tired. We now know how and why these invaders are wreaking havoc on our overall health and well-being. As promised, I will now share with you the different ways we can combat these offenders. To do so, we must repair and rebuild the organs needed to remove these toxins from our bodies. The cornerstones to this objective are a healthy and well-functioning liver and gut.

I must again emphasize that, before starting any new diet, taking supplements, or making significant changes to your lifestyle, it is important to consult with your health-care provider. The information and advice provided in this book are not intended to replace professional medical consultation, diagnosis, or treatment. Your doctor can provide personalized advice based on your health history and current medical condition to ensure any new dietary changes or supplements are safe and appropriate for you.

CHAPTER TEN:

Repairing the Liver: A Key Organ in Detoxification

With our battle against endocrine-disrupting chemicals (EDCs), the liver emerges as a pivotal organ, diligently working to detoxify our bodies from numerous pollutants we may encounter every day. Understanding the profound role of the liver in detoxification will help us appreciate the need to nurture its health. Renewing and strengthening our liver health can be a potent strategy in reducing the impacts of EDCs.

As part of the many detoxifications processes that are executed by the liver, a systematic, three-phase system is used to neutralize and eliminate toxins, including EDCs, from our bodies. Each phase is integral and relies on different enzymatic and biochemical processes to ensure that harmful substances are adequately addressed and removed.

Let's think of your liver like a massive, 24-7 international airport terminal; but instead of travelers, it's processing thousands of chemicals, toxins, drugs, and hormones that enter your body every day. To prevent these "chemical passengers" from entering your body's circulation unchecked, the liver runs them through a three-phase security checkpoint system.

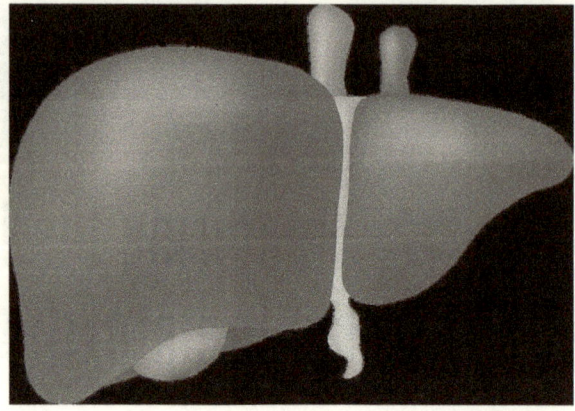
CC BY 4.0

During phase one, the liver performs the ID check and initial screening. Just like at the airport where a security guard scans your ID and luggage, a group of enzymes called cytochrome P450 screen the incoming passengers.

- These enzymes chemically modify toxins by breaking them down into intermediates (often more reactive or unstable than when in their original form). These byproducts can often be more dangerous than the original toxins, so they need to be quickly neutralized in the next phase before they cause damage.
- Think of this like opening someone's luggage and finding suspicious items that now need extra attention.

During phase two, the liver then performs a neutralizing process called conjugation. Now that the dangerous passengers have been flagged, phase two steps in like a team of customs agents who handcuff the suspicious travelers and bag their dangerous items.

- This phase adds a "tag" or molecule (like sulfur, glycine, or glutathione) to the toxin to neutralize it and make it water-soluble.

- This is called conjugation, and it helps prepare the toxin for safe removal. The end result is that the once-reactive toxin is now rendered harmless and ready to be escorted out of the terminal.

During phase three, the liver transports and eliminates the toxins. This final phase is like guiding the flagged unruly, dangerous—but now neutralized—passengers to the exit gate for departure.

- The liver hands these compounds over to transport proteins that ship them out using either airport security staff (which we will call bile) or FBI agents (which, in this scenario, are the kidneys). The bile gets the toxins out through the intestines via stool while the kidneys kick them out through urine.
- This is where detoxification is completed, and the body finally says goodbye to the harmful chemicals.

If you're overloaded with toxins from EDCs, alcohol, or processed foods—or lack the right "detox crew" nutrients like B vitamins, glutathione, and magnesium—then the airport gets overwhelmed and the whole system backs up.

- Phase one runs too fast, producing toxic byproducts that are more dangerous than the original toxins.
- Phase two can't keep up with neutralization due to a lack of nutrients.
- Phase three exits are blocked due to constipation, dehydration, or kidney issues.

The disastrous result is that the airport gets run over with terrorists, and the bad passengers start wandering the terminals again, causing inflammation, fatigue, hormonal imbalance, and even disease. When no reinforcements are sent and this is left unchecked, the airport ultimately shuts down. Let's dig deeper.

Three Phases of Liver Detoxification

Phase One: Biotransformation of Toxins
This first phase breaks down toxins.
- **Enzymatic action:** This phase utilizes a set of enzymes, primarily cytochrome P450 enzymes, to initiate the breakdown of toxins.
- **Conversion to intermediates:** Since EDCs are often lipophilic (fat-soluble) toxins, they need to be converted into more polar intermediates by introducing or exposing a functional group, rendering them more water-soluble. The more water-soluble the toxin, the more easily it can be excreted.
- **Free radicals:** During this phase, while toxins are being broken down, free radicals are generated. This makes antioxidants crucial for combating potential oxidative stress from the free radicals. Therefore, the more that free radicals are generated in your body, the more the liver becomes overwhelmed to remove these toxins from your body.

Phase Two: Conjugation
This second phase neutralizes toxins.
- **Synergizing with phase one:** The by-products from phase one are further neutralized through conjugation with molecules like glutathione, sulfate, or glycine, which enhances their water solubility.
- **Neutralization:** This step effectively neutralizes the reactive compounds, preventing them from causing cellular damage.
- **Enhancing excretion:** The increased solubility facilitates their excretion via bile or urine.

Phase Three: Transport and Elimination

This third phase eliminates toxins.

- **Cellular transporters:** This phase employs cellular transport proteins to pump the now neutralized and conjugated toxins out of the liver cells.
- **Excretion pathways:** The toxins are directed toward the appropriate excretory pathways, typically via the bile into the stool or via the kidneys into the urine.
- **Comprehensive elimination:** Ensuring efficient functionality in this phase is important to prevent reabsorption of toxins and ensure they are fully removed from the body.

To further illustrate this, I have included the diagram below, showing the three phases of liver detoxification with a list of essential nutrients needed to support each process. You can imagine that if you are deficient in many of those nutrients, your detoxification by the liver will be compromised. The second image depicts how fat-soluble toxins like EDCs, alcohol, pesticides, and food additives enter the liver for detoxification and are converted into water-soluble byproducts ready for elimination in the stool or in the urine. Any disruption to any of these phases can lead to toxins being stored as fat rather than being eliminated.

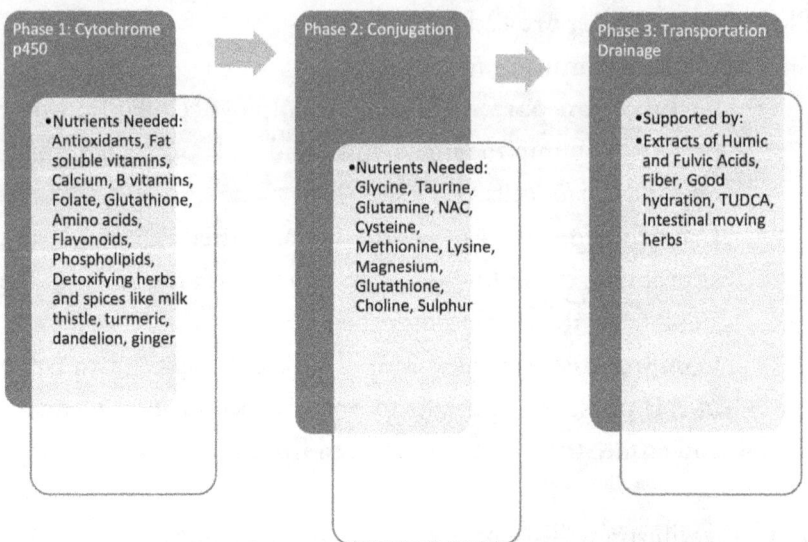

This Photo by Unknown Author is licensed under CC BY-SA

Supporting Each Phase: A Targeted Approach

Given the meticulous progression through these phases, supporting each phase of liver detoxification with the proper nutrients is paramount for our defense.

For Phase I: Antioxidants like vitamins C and E, selenium, fat-soluble vitamins like vitamin D, glutathione, B vitamins, and phytochemicals from cruciferous vegetables can combat oxidative stress generated during this phase. It can be supported by using detoxifying herbs like milk thistle, turmeric, dandelion, and ginger.

For Phase II: Sufficient protein intake and sulfur-containing foods like garlic and sulfur-containing vegetables provide glucosinolate. Amino acids like glycine, glutamine, cysteine, taurine, and lysine are the building blocks for proteins. The antioxidant glutathione also supports this phase.

For Phase III: Adequate fiber ensures the bound toxins are escorted out of the body, and maintaining optimal kidney function supports urinary excretion. The addition of minerals like humic and fulvic acids can maintain this phase. The addition of bile acids like tauroursodeoxycholic acid (TUDCA) can promote healthy bile flow.

The Liver: A Detoxification Powerhouse
- **Role in metabolism:** Beyond its numerous metabolic functions, the liver is essential in detoxifying harmful substances, including EDCs, from our bodies.
- **Biotransformation of toxins:** Through a three-phase detoxification process, the liver transforms toxins into less-harmful substances that can be safely excreted.
- **Vitality and resilience:** Ensuring liver health is paramount for metabolic balance, hormone regulation, and fostering resilience against environmental toxins.

The Assault of EDCs on Liver Function
- **Toxic burden:** Prolonged exposure to EDCs can overwhelm the liver's detoxification capacity, potentially leading to impaired function.
- **Metabolic disruption:** EDCs can disrupt liver metabolism, hindering its capability to effectively regulate glucose and lipid homeostasis.
- **Oxidative stress:** Many EDCs induce oxidative stress, which might impair liver cells and jeopardize liver health.

Strategies to Uphold Liver Health
- **Nutritional support:** Opt for foods rich in antioxidants (e.g., berries, nuts, vegetables) to combat oxidative stress. Include cruciferous vegetables that support phase two of liver detoxification. Incorporate foods high in fiber to facilitate the excretion of detoxified substances.

- **Hydration:** Ensure adequate water intake to assist the liver in flushing out toxins and supporting metabolic processes.
- **Avoidance of additional toxins:** Limit alcohol consumption, and be mindful of medications that may increase the liver's workload.

Holistic Approaches to Liver Health
- **Herbal allies:** Milk thistle, turmeric, artichoke extract, and dandelion are widely recognized for their potential to support liver function and health.
- **Mindful practices:** Manage stress through mindfulness practices like meditation or yoga, considering the indirect impacts of stress on liver health.

The Bigger Picture: Lifestyle and Environment
- **Reducing EDC exposure:** Be mindful of sources of EDC exposure, including plastics, cosmetics, and pesticides, and seek safer alternatives whenever possible.
- **Creating a healthy living environment:** Consider air purifiers, and choose household products that are free from harmful chemicals.

Leveraging Scientific Knowledge
- **Staying informed:** Keep abreast of ongoing research on EDCs and liver health to adapt strategies accordingly.
- **Community involvement:** Engage in and promote community efforts aimed at reducing widespread EDC exposure.

Conclusion

The liver, in its silent diligence, plays a crucial role in our battle against the pervasive threat of EDCs. By merging scientific knowledge, holistic practices, and mindful living, we can strengthen this vital organ, thereby safeguarding our metabolic health and reducing the toxic burden in our bodies. The pursuit to understand and protect our liver is not merely a personal journey but is intrinsically linked with global efforts toward reducing EDCs in our environment, ultimately paving the path toward collective health and well-being.

Scan to learn more about the liver.

All videos are provided courtesy of Alilia Medical Media. Copying and/or downloading of any of the videos or animations to any social media platforms such as YouTube, Facebook, or TikTok is strictly prohibited.

©Alila Medical Media. All medical materials are for information purposes *only* and are *not* intended to be medical advice.

CHAPTER ELEVEN:

Healing the Gut: Restoring Gut Health to Combat EDC Effects

Gut health is an essential factor in our overall well-being, influencing everything from our immune system to our mental health. Moreover, a healthy gut can be an ardent defense against the insidious influences of endocrine-disrupting chemicals (EDCs). As EDCs potentially impair gut function and microbiome balance, formulating strategies to restore and maintain adequate gut health is valuable in limiting the harmful impacts of these pervasive chemicals.

Your gut is like a beautiful garden teeming with life. The soil is your gut lining (intestinal wall and mucosal layer) that acts as the foundation to support microbial life, absorb nutrients, and communicate with the immune and endocrine systems. The gardeners, bees, and worms are the helpful good bacteria (probiotics) that tend the soil, manage the weeds, and produce healthy compounds. The plants are the nutrients, hormones, neurotransmitters, and enzymes that grow or are produced by gut activity, especially by the good microbes. This garden feeds you—literally and figuratively—by helping to digest food, regulate hormones, produce neurotransmitters, and maintain your immune system.

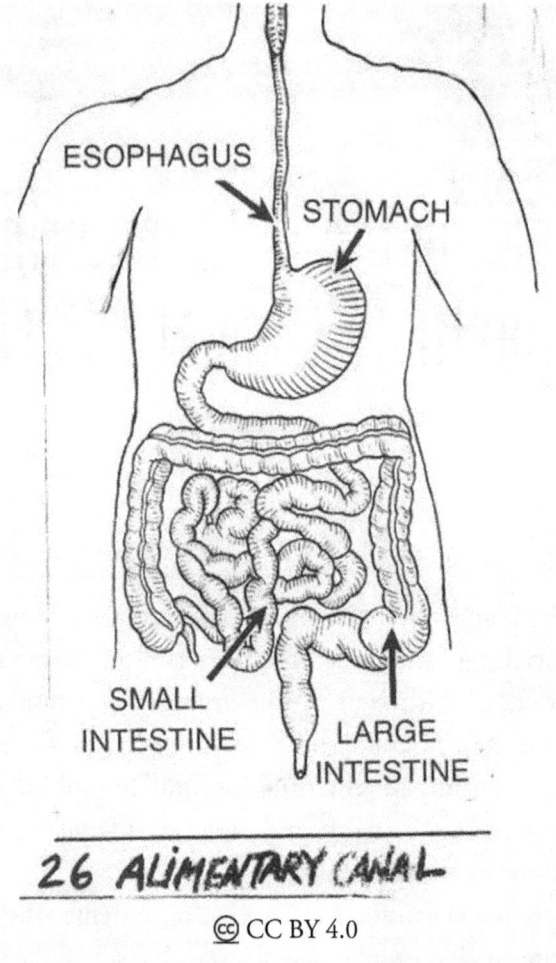

26 ALIMENTARY CANAL

CC BY 4.0

A healthy diet, proper hydration, and lifestyle habits (including adequate sleep, exercise, and eating fiber-rich foods) act like the water and sunshine that nourish the garden. The bad bacteria are like weeds or pests that steal nutrients, damage plants (hormonal pathways), cause inflammation, and create toxic byproducts. A healthy garden has the right balance between good and bad microbes—this balance is known as eubiosis. The opposite of eubiosis is dysbiosis, which refers to an imbalance or disruption in the microbial community.

Now picture someone spraying the garden with an invisible chemical mist, which represents those nasty endocrine-disrupting chemicals (EDCs). EDCs from plastics, pesticides, personal care products, or food packaging seep into the garden soil (your gut lining). These toxic substances act like herbicides and synthetic fertilizers, wiping out beneficial microbes and disturbing the soil structure. They kill or suppress good bacteria, feed the bad bacteria, increase intestinal permeability (a.k.a. "leaky gut") and interfere with gut hormone signaling (GLP-1, PYY, and serotonin). When EDCs (like BPA or phthalates) enter the gut, they damage the soil (gut lining), killing off good microbes and altering the absorption and protection systems.

While the balance in the gut is disrupted, good microbes are outnumbered and harmful bacteria start multiplying. This leads to weeds growing unchecked and inflammation spreading like wildfires. Weeds (bad bacteria) overtake the garden, reducing the production of healthy plants (hormones like GLP-1 and serotonin). The garden stops yielding nutritious produce such as neurotransmitters and gut hormones.

This abnormal shift in the balance between good and bad bacteria is called dysbiosis, and it creates the perfect storm. This imbalance in the gut leads to symptoms of bloating, constipation, irritable bowel syndrome, food cravings, weight gain, and fatigue. In addition, mood disorders, due to less serotonin and dopamine production, can occur. Since over 70 percent of the immune system lives in the gut, a dysfunctional gut can also lead to weakened immunity.

Fortunately for us, the gut is resilient. Like a garden, it can heal with the proper care and attention. Before we review solutions on how to restore your gut, let's learn more.

Understanding the Impact of EDCs on Gut Health

Microbiome disruption: EDCs can alter the composition and function of gut microbiota, potentially leading to dysbiosis, which is associated with various health issues like obesity, immune dysfunction, and even neurodevelopmental disorders.

Polychlorinated biphenyls (PCBs) are a class of EDCs that have been identified to disrupt gut microbiota and increase gut permeability. The complexity of the gut biome can be negatively affected by PCBs in a manner that compromises metabolic health and immune function. Studies have shown that PCB exposure can alter the composition of the gut microbiome, reducing the abundance of good bacteria and enabling the proliferation of pathogenic or bad bacteria, leading to gut dysbiosis.

Immune response: This alteration in gut permeability can also instigate an immune response, as the leaked substances are identified as foreign invaders by the body's immune system, thereby elevating inflammatory markers and possibly leading to chronic, low-grade inflammation.

PCBs can also induce inflammation within the gut by increasing intestinal permeability and allowing harmful substances to leak into the bloodstream.

Gut permeability: There's evidence that EDCs may increase intestinal permeability, sometimes referred to as "leaky gut," which allows toxins and undigested food particles to enter the bloodstream, triggering inflammation and immune responses.

PCBs have been shown to enhance gut permeability by disrupting the tight junctions that regulate intestinal barrier function. This enhanced permeability allows toxins, microbes, and undigested food particles to escape into the bloodstream, prompting systemic inflammation and potentially contributing to various health issues.

The diagram below depicts the differences between a healthy and unhealthy (or "leaky") gut. Chronic exposure to stress, toxins, and chemicals can cause our normal barriers to weaken, allowing them to penetrate and enter our bloodstream.

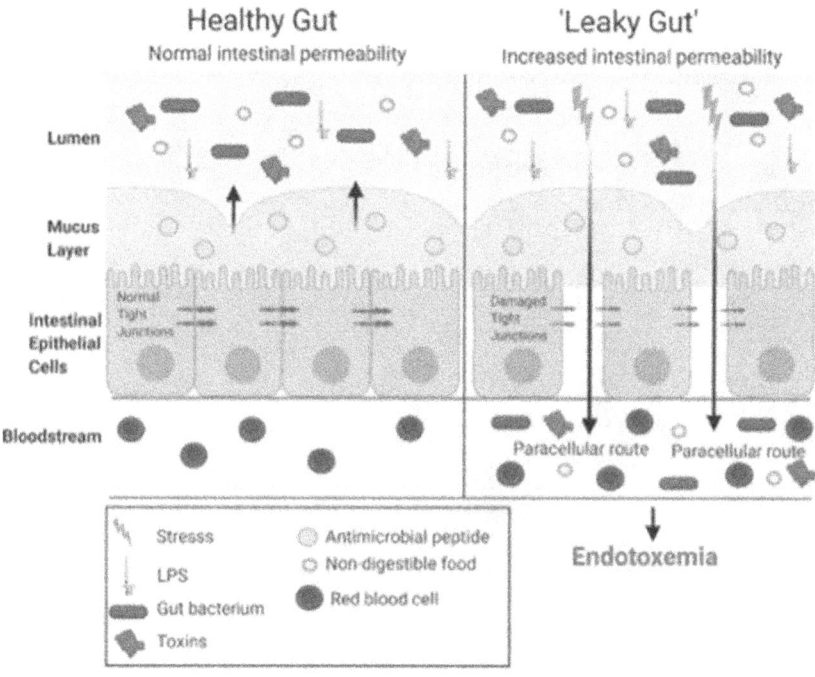

This Photo by Unknown Author is licensed under CC BY

Strategies for Gut Restoration and Protection

Within this section, as we review strategies for gut restoration and protection, it's important to know how to reduce PCB exposure and neutralize its effects, particularly in the context of gut health. When exploring strategies like nourishing the microbiome with probiotics and prebiotics, and replenishing and repairing the gut lining with healing foods, such interventions must be reviewed and approved by your primary care provider.

Due to the widespread presence of PCBs, strategies aimed at supporting liver detoxification, as was discussed in the last chapter, should accompany strategies to improve the gut as a dual approach. A well-functioning gut enhances the liver's abilities to detoxify and excrete these toxicants.

1. Nourishing the Microbiome

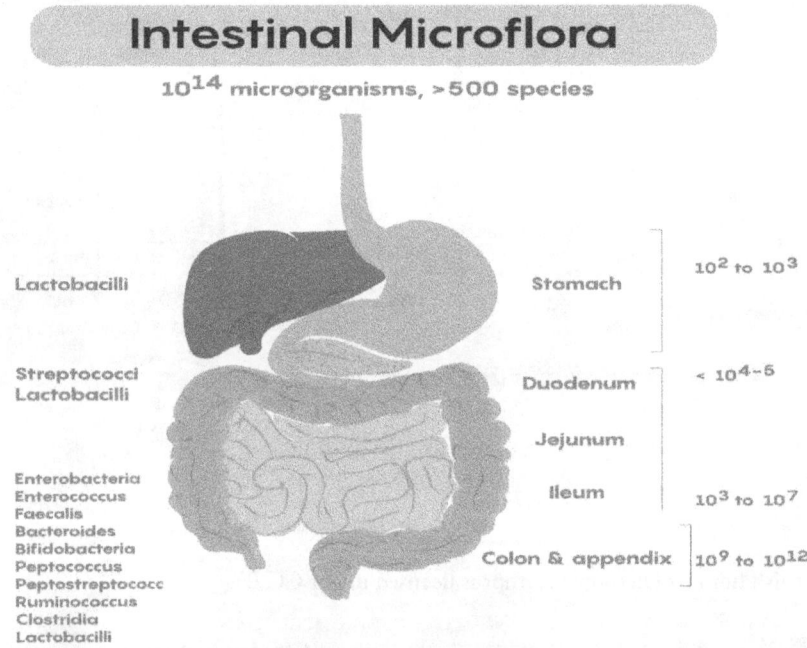

This Photo by Unknown Author is licensed under CC BY

Probiotics: We must replant the garden with beneficial strains. Incorporate fermented foods like yogurt, kefir, sauerkraut, kimchi, and kombucha or high-quality supplements to bolster beneficial gut bacteria.

Prebiotics: We need to feed our garden by feeding our good bacteria. Fuel beneficial bacteria with fibrous foods such as garlic, onions, and asparagus, and resistant starches like green bananas and cooked and cooled potatoes.

2. Replenishing and Repairing the Gut Lining

Bone broth: Rich in collagen and gelatin, bone broth can be soothing and reparative for the gut lining.

L-glutamine: This amino acid plays a crucial role in repairing and maintaining the integrity of the intestinal wall.

3. Reducing Inflammation

Anti-inflammatory foods: Prioritize foods rich in omega-3, like fatty fish and flaxseeds, and antioxidant-rich berries and leafy greens to combat inflammation. Adding whole, unprocessed foods like fruits, vegetables, and lean proteins provides essential nutrients and fiber crucial for gut health.

Elimination diet: Identify and remove potential food sensitivities and allergens, which could be contributing to gut issues and inflammation. We must remove toxins by minimizing our exposure to EDCs found in our food, water, plastics, and personal care products. It is recommended to reduce your intake of ultra-processed foods, artificial sweeteners, and excessive sugar, all of which negatively impact the gut microbiome.

4. Supporting Detoxification

Fiber: Ensure a high intake of fiber from fruits, vegetables, legumes, and whole grains to bind to toxins and facilitate their excretion.

Hydration: Just like you need to keep your soil moist in the garden, so too must you keep your gut hydrated. Adequate water intake supports detoxification and promotes healthy bowel movements.

Tending the garden daily requires us to embrace a gut-friendly lifestyle.

Manage stress: Practices like mindfulness, meditation, yoga, and deep-breathing exercises can help manage stress levels, which are inherently linked to gut health.

Restorative sleep: Ensuring seven to nine hours of adequate-quality sleep per night supports overall health, including gut function.

Movement: Regular, moderate-intensity exercise can foster a healthy gut by promoting motility and a favorable microbiome.

Addressing stress management, sufficient sleep, and regular exercise becomes even more critical in the context of EDC and PCB exposure, as these lifestyle factors can significantly modulate immune function, inflammation, and gut health, providing additional defenses against the deceptive impacts of such chemicals.

In navigating through a world permeated by EDCs, preserving our gut health becomes not only a method of defense but a winning attack in the war against a toxic environment. Ensuring our gut is supported, nurtured, and protected is key to a program aimed at minimizing EDC impacts on our bodies.

CHAPTER TWELVE:

Go Green with Clean Food as Medicine: Optimal Nutrition to Counteract EDCs

The food we consume plays a significant role in determining our overall health and well-being. In a world where endocrine-disrupting chemicals (EDCs) permeate, making conscientious food choices becomes not just a matter of nourishing our bodies, but also a significant strategy in minimizing the exposure and impacts of these harmful chemicals. This chapter outlines the profound connection between our dietary habits and the body's susceptibility to EDCs, providing insight into adopting a "green," clean, and medicinal approach to eating.

Choosing Organic: A Great Ally Against EDCs

Organic foods have gained great attention as a great option to reduce the intake of EDCs. Pesticides, herbicides, and synthetic fertilizers—common culprits of endocrine disruption—are less likely to contaminate organic produce. Consuming organic foods, when possible, can be a proactive step toward limiting the ingestion of EDCs and supporting the body's natural detoxification processes.

Embracing organic foods is a fundamental strategy in reducing the risks associated with EDC exposure through diet. Eating organic produce, grown without the use of synthetic pesticides, herbicides, and fertilizers, substantially reduces the influx of these disruptive chemicals into our bodies. When it comes to certain fruits and vegetables that tend to harbor higher pesticide residues, opting for organic versions can be profoundly impactful.

One significant resource to guide our organic food choices is the concept of the Dirty Dozen. This term refers to a list of twelve fruits and vegetables that have been found to contain the highest levels of pesticide residues. By prioritizing organic versions of these items, we can strategically minimize our pesticide exposure.

The Dirty Dozen typically includes the following:
- Strawberries
- Spinach
- Kale, collard, and mustard greens
- Nectarines
- Apples
- Grapes
- Cherries
- Peaches
- Pears
- Bell peppers and hot peppers
- Celery
- Tomatoes

While incorporating organic produce is a potent approach, it's also advisable to balance this with overall dietary variety and nutritional intake. Therefore, the absence of organic options should not deter the consumption of fruits and vegetables altogether. Awareness and discernment, backed by resources such as the Dirty Dozen, enable more empowered and health-conscious choices in our journey toward mitigating the impacts of EDCs.

Phytonutrients: Natural Detoxifiers

Incorporating a rainbow of fruits and vegetables in the diet augments the intake of phytonutrients—natural compounds with potent antioxidant and anti-inflammatory properties. These phytonutrients can assist in mitigating the oxidative stress and inflammation facilitated by EDCs, supporting cellular health and resilience.

Cruciferous Vegetables: Allies of the Endocrine System

Cruciferous vegetables like broccoli, brussels sprouts, and kale possess specific compounds such as sulforaphane, known for their protective effects on the endocrine system. They may help in modulating estrogen metabolism and enhancing the body's defense mechanisms against hormone-disrupting chemicals. If, however, you have thyroid disease, it is best to consume cruciferous vegetables cooked rather than raw.

Fiber-Rich Foods: Supporting Gut Health and Detoxification

A diet abundant in fiber-rich foods such as whole grains, legumes, fruits, and vegetables supports a healthy gut microbiome, a key player in detoxification pathways. Fiber aids in promoting bowel regularity, facilitating the excretion of toxins and EDCs from the body.

Healthy Fats: Modulating Inflammation

Incorporating sources of omega-3 fatty acids like flaxseeds, walnuts, and fatty fish can help modulate the inflammation induced by EDC exposure. These fats also play a role in supporting cellular integrity and overall hormonal balance.

Hydration: Enhancing Elimination of Toxins

Proper hydration is fundamental in promoting the body's natural detoxification processes. It assists in optimizing kidney function and aiding in the efficient elimination of waste products and various toxins, including EDCs.

Mindful Consumption: Limiting Processed Foods and Plastics

Minimizing the consumption of heavily processed and packaged foods can help in reducing exposure to EDCs commonly found in food packaging materials. Adopting mindful practices such as using glass or stainless-steel containers, avoiding heating food in plastic containers, and being cautious of canned foods lined with BPA are practical steps toward limiting EDC exposure.

The key to improving our bodies' defenses against EDCs is maintaining an anti-inflammatory diet. The best anti-inflammatory foods to include in your arsenal are the following:

1. **Garlic** boasts antibacterial, antiviral, and antioxidant properties and can be eaten as one raw clove per day or added to many foods like soups, veggies, and meats.
2. **Ginger** prevents the production of cytokines (proteins that trigger chronic inflammation), improves digestion, and can reduce cholesterol and blood sugar levels.
3. **Cruciferous vegetables like broccoli, cabbage, and cauliflower** are high in potassium, magnesium, and sulforaphane which can lower oxidative stress and reduce risk of developing cancer.

4. **Olive oil** is rich in heart-healthy fatty acids, antioxidants, and polyphenols. It can be taken as a shot every morning or drizzled liberally over foods.
5. **Berries** are high in antioxidants called flavonoids that reduce free-radical damage to cells and can help fight cancer. Eat at least one cup daily.
6. **Turmeric** is the revered spice in Indian culture and is touted for its anti-inflammatory benefits with arthritis, cancer, and even Alzheimer's disease. It can be taken as a supplement or cooked in many dishes.
7. **Bone broth** is full of calcium, magnesium, and glucosamine needed for gut repair, joints, and collagen production for skin, hair, and nails. Sip a cup a day, or add to soups or to quinoa for added flavor and health benefits.
8. **Coconut oil** is a saturated fat. If used in moderation, it can increase fat metabolism, weight loss, and digestion.
9. **Cinnamon** is proven to reduce sugars and protect against oxidative stress. You can add it to your morning coffee or to cereal, oatmeal, or yogurt.
10. **Moringa** is hailed as the "tree of life" or "miracle tree" for its vast medicinal and nutritional benefits such as lowering cholesterol, decreasing inflammation, and reducing blood sugars.
11. **Leafy greens like spinach and kale** are rich in flavonoids, vitamin K, vitamin C, and potassium which are essential for reducing free radicals and oxidative stress.
12. **Fatty fish** is high in omega-3 fatty acids and B vitamins needed for cellular repair. Increase your intake of salmon, tuna, and herring to three ounces twice a week.
13. **Chia seeds** are high in fiber, protein, and omega-3 fatty acids, and they have been shown to reduce blood pressure, lower cholesterol,

and reverse inflammation. They can be added to pancakes and smoothies or made as chia pudding.
14. **Select nuts, like almonds and walnuts,** are high in fiber and protein, which makes them great snacks to keep hunger at bay. They can be added to salads or yogurt.
15. **Beets** are high in an amino acid called betaine which helps with acid reflux and helps protect the body from environmental stressors. Numerous studies show its beneficial effects in lowering blood pressure, increasing energy levels, and improving blood flow to the brain.

We must also avoid the most inflammatory foods. These include the following:
1. **Processed or packaged foods** are full of saturated fats, preservatives, and chemicals. Examples are hot dogs, lunch meat, bacon, sausage, meal kits, deli meats, prepackaged meals, fast foods, and most items within the inner grocery aisles.
2. **Fried foods** are usually cooked in unhealthy saturated or trans-saturated fatty oils which increase production of advanced glycation end products (AGEs) and inflammatory omega-6 fatty acids. Pan-seared or baked foods are healthier alternatives.
3. **Sugary beverages** such as sodas, sports drinks, energy drinks, and juices can be loaded with high-fructose syrup or artificial sweeteners that lead to increased inflammatory markers. Switch to green or black teas sweetened with monk fruit or stevia.
4. **White bread and white rice** have been stripped of their fiber and nutrients, leaving them high in carbohydrates which cause spikes in blood sugars. Consider changing to quinoa, brown rice, or sweet potatoes as alternatives.
5. **Packaged baked goods** such as boxed cookies, crackers, chips, muffins, pastries, bread and cakes are full of partially hydrogenated

oils which contain trans-fatty acids that have been shown to increase heart disease.
6. **Flavored yogurts** are often confused as a healthy product, but unfortunately, they are full of sugar. Opt for plain Greek yogurt and add fresh fruit instead.
7. **Margarine** has been found to be higher in saturated fats than butter and contains trans fats linked with systemic inflammation and heart disease. Choose olive oil or avocado oil instead.
8. **Processed cheeses** were found to have high amounts of saturated fats. Swap American cheese with natural cheeses like feta or mozzarella cheese.
9. **Cereals and granolas** are high in refined starches and sugars that cause inflammation. Select better choices such as eggs, yogurt, or high-fiber smoothies for breakfast.
10. **Grilled and BBQ foods**, when cooked at extremely high temperatures, can release inflammatory advanced glycation end products (AGEs) that have been linked with cancer. Marinating foods in an acidic solution like vinegar or lemon juice before cooking can cut AGEs in half.

Intermittent Fasting and Its Role in Combating Exposure to Endocrine-Disrupting Chemicals (EDCs)

Endocrine-disrupting chemicals (EDCs) are compounds found in many everyday products and environmental sources, including plastics, personal care items, pesticides, and even food packaging. These chemicals interfere with the endocrine system, leading to hormonal imbalances, weight gain, insulin resistance, and other metabolic issues. Some common EDCs include bisphenol A (BPA), phthalates, and polychlorinated biphenyls (PCBs).

Intermittent fasting (IF) is a dietary pattern that alternates between periods of eating and fasting. Research suggests that intermittent fasting can offer several benefits that may help decrease some of the harmful effects of EDC exposure. Here's how intermittent fasting may support detoxification and combat the adverse health effects of EDCs:

1. **Enhancing Autophagy and Cellular Repair**
   - **What Is Autophagy?**
     » Autophagy is a natural cellular process where cells "clean out" damaged components, including dysfunctional proteins and organelles, allowing for cellular repair and regeneration. This process is pivotal for removing toxic substances and cellular waste, including compounds that may have been damaged or altered by EDC exposure.
   - **Intermittent Fasting and Autophagy**
     » Fasting triggers autophagy, especially during prolonged periods without food (typically sixteen hours or more). This cellular "cleanup" mechanism can help cells remove damaged materials and may reduce the toxic load accumulated from EDCs. By enhancing autophagy, intermittent fasting may support cellular resilience against the damaging effects of these chemicals.

2. **Improving Insulin Sensitivity and Glucose Metabolism**
   - **EDCs and Insulin Resistance**
     » Many EDCs, including BPA and phthalates, have been shown to interfere with glucose metabolism and lead to insulin resistance, a precursor to obesity and type 2 diabetes. EDCs can mimic or disrupt hormonal pathways that regulate glucose uptake, leading to metabolic imbalances.
   - **Intermittent Fasting's Role**
     » Intermittent fasting (IF) has been shown to improve insulin sensitivity and support better glucose regulation

by reducing insulin levels and promoting fat metabolism. By reducing insulin resistance, IF can prevent some of the metabolic disruptions caused by EDC exposure. Lower insulin levels also mean less fat storage, which can help reduce the bioaccumulation of fat-soluble EDCs stored in adipose tissue.

3. **Supporting Weight Loss and Reducing Fat Stores**
   - **EDCs and Fat Accumulation**
     » Certain EDCs, known as obesogens, promote fat accumulation and weight gain. These chemicals disrupt the normal hormonal signals involved in fat storage, leading to increased adiposity. Since EDCs are often stored in body fat, excess body fat can lead to a higher accumulation and prolonged exposure to these toxins.
   - **Intermittent Fasting and Fat Loss**
     » Intermittent fasting promotes weight loss by increasing fat metabolism and reducing overall calorie intake. As fat stores decrease, so does the body's reservoir for storing EDCs, which could help reduce the overall toxic load. By facilitating fat loss, IF can help lower the body's burden of fat-soluble EDCs stored in adipose tissue.

4. **Reducing Oxidative Stress and Inflammation**
   - **EDCs and Inflammatory Response**
     » Exposure to EDCs can lead to oxidative stress and chronic low-grade inflammation, which contribute to various health issues, including metabolic syndrome, cardiovascular disease, and even cancer. EDCs interfere with the balance of free radicals and antioxidants in the body, leading to cellular damage.

- **Antioxidant Benefits of Fasting**
  » Fasting has been shown to reduce oxidative stress and inflammation by lowering pro-inflammatory markers and supporting antioxidant production. By reducing oxidative stress, intermittent fasting helps protect cells from EDC-induced damage. In addition, the reduction in inflammation supports overall immune health and helps the body's natural defense mechanisms respond more readily to toxic exposure.

5. Hormone Regulation and Balancing Endocrine Health
   - **EDCs and Hormonal Disruptions**
     » EDCs interfere with hormonal balance by mimicking or blocking the actions of natural hormones like estrogen, testosterone, and thyroid hormones. This disruption can lead to conditions such as estrogen dominance, thyroid dysfunction, and reproductive issues.
   - **Fasting's Effect on Hormones**
     » Intermittent fasting has been shown to help regulate hormones involved in metabolism, stress, and appetite. By supporting balanced levels of insulin, growth hormone, and other metabolic hormones, IF can help counter some of the hormonal imbalances induced by EDCs. This balancing effect may help mitigate the impact of EDCs on hormonal health.

6. Promoting Detoxification Through Increased Mitochondrial Function
   - **Mitochondrial Health and EDCs**
     » EDCs have been shown to impair the function of mitochondria, the energy-producing centers of cells, which can lead to decreased cellular energy and compromised

detoxification. Mitochondria are crucial for breaking down and processing toxic compounds, and healthy mitochondrial function supports overall detoxification.
- **Intermittent Fasting and Mitochondrial Efficiency**
  » Fasting promotes mitochondrial biogenesis, which is the process of creating new, healthy mitochondria. By boosting mitochondrial function, intermittent fasting helps the body efficiently detoxify and process potentially harmful substances, including EDCs.

7. **Supporting Liver Health for Detoxification**
   - **Role of the Liver in Detoxifying EDCs**
     » The liver is the body's primary detox organ and plays a critical role in processing and eliminating EDCs. However, chronic exposure to EDCs can overload the liver, impairing its ability to effectively detoxify the body.
   - **Fasting and Liver Function**
     » Intermittent fasting can support liver health by giving the digestive system regular rest periods, allowing the liver to focus on detoxification rather than constant food processing. This rest period may allow the liver to break down and excrete toxins more efficiently, helping to clear EDCs from the body.

Practical Tips for Implementing Intermittent Fasting to Combat EDC Exposure

1. **Start with a Simple Protocol**
   » Beginners can start with the 16/8 method, fasting for sixteen hours and eating within an eight-hour window. This is one of the easiest ways to introduce intermittent fasting while allowing the body to trigger autophagy and support metabolic health.

2. **Stay Hydrated**
   » Drink plenty of water during your fasting period to support kidney function and help flush out toxins. Herbal teas and electrolyte supplements can also aid in detoxification without breaking your fast.
3. **Incorporate Nutrient-Dense Foods During Eating Windows**
   » Focus on foods rich in antioxidants, healthy fats, fiber, and lean protein to support liver function, reduce inflammation, and enhance cellular repair. Foods like leafy greens, berries, turmeric, and fatty fish are excellent choices for combating oxidative stress and inflammation associated with EDC exposure.
4. **Avoid Processed Foods and Sugar**
   » Processed foods and refined sugars can increase oxidative stress, inflammation, and insulin resistance. These foods also contain additives and preservatives that may add to your toxic load, undermining the benefits of fasting.

Scan to learn more about intermittent fasting.

All videos are provided courtesy of Alilia Medical Media. Copying and/or downloading of any of the videos or animations to any social media platforms such as YouTube, Facebook, or TikTok is strictly prohibited.

©Alila Medical Media. All medical materials are for information purposes *only* and are *not* intended to be medical advice.

Conclusion

Empowering ourselves with knowledge and making informed food choices are instrumental in navigating the pervasive presence of EDCs in our environment. Adopting a nutritional approach that emphasizes organic, wholesome, and nourishing foods not only fosters overall health but also fortifies the body's resilience against the detrimental impacts of endocrine disruptors. In embracing the philosophy that food is medicine, we unveil a powerful strategy in our arsenal against the invisible onslaught of EDCs.

Intermittent fasting is a powerful tool that can support your body in combating the harmful effects of EDC exposure. By enhancing autophagy, promoting fat loss, reducing oxidative stress, improving insulin sensitivity, and supporting liver and mitochondrial function, intermittent fasting helps reduce the toxic load and balances hormonal health. Adopting intermittent fasting as part of a healthy lifestyle may offer a natural way to mitigate the risks associated with EDCs and support overall well-being.

Always consult a health-care provider before starting intermittent fasting, especially if you have any medical conditions or concerns.

CHAPTER THIRTEEN:

How to Reduce Obesogens Naturally

If you're like me, you've probably had countless frustrating moments during your weight loss journey. I, too, followed my diet religiously, did my yoga, and even cut out all carbs, sweets, and alcohol. I would see an initial loss of six pounds only to see a plateau and later regain. Oh, the agony! I never thought that toxins hiding in my fat cells could be the culprit preventing my success toward a healthy weight. Even more appalling is the fact that when we restrict our calories and begin to lose weight, the levels of circulating toxins can actually increase above our pre-weight loss levels. As we detox and release those toxins, they can redistribute and make their homes in other fatty tissues like those in the liver. Remember, fatty toxins are attracted to fatty tissues. This explains the alarmingly increasing rates of fatty liver disease. Thus, a vicious cycle plays in the background preventing us from properly excreting these chemicals, leading to a decreased fat-burning ability, reduced metabolism, and low energy levels. Fear not, my friends. I'm here to encourage you to realize that we can fight back. In every war, we need a battle plan to attack in a more strategic and precise way.

This is why I spent so much time focusing on how to repair the liver and gut. The key is that, in addition to having a well-functioning liver that neutralizes the toxins, we also need a well-functioning gut and kidney to remove them from our bodies and avoid accumulating again.

In chapter seven, I outlined a detailed review of the different pathways by which EDCs lead to hormone disruptions and thereby cause obesity. Now let us target those ten pathways contributing to obesity, focusing on how natural methods can help reduce the impact of obesogens—chemicals that promote fat accumulation and disrupt metabolic processes. By addressing each pathway (hypothalamus, pituitary gland, thyroid gland, gut, stomach, liver, pancreas, adrenal glands, reproductive organs, and fat cells), you can support a healthier hormonal balance, improve your metabolism, and reduce your risk of weight gain.

1. **Hypothalamus (Appetite Control)**
   - **Avoid high-fructose corn syrup and processed foods:** These can stimulate appetite by disrupting leptin signaling in the hypothalamus, leading to overeating.
   - **Include omega-3 fatty acids:** Omega-3s found in fatty fish, flaxseed, and walnuts can help improve leptin sensitivity and reduce inflammation, which supports hypothalamic health.
   - **Limit exposure to artificial sweeteners:** Some studies suggest artificial sweeteners can interfere with hunger signaling and contribute to increased appetite. Opt for natural sweeteners like stevia or monk fruit in moderation.
   - **Get at least ten to fifteen minutes of unfiltered sunlight in the morning:** This boosts melatonin. Another way to boost natural melatonin is by eating pistachios, sardines, goji berries, and mushrooms.

- Citrus scents such as grapefruit have been shown to reduce appetite.
- **Herbs and Supplements**
  » **Green tea extract** contains catechins that help regulate hunger hormones and can enhance fat burning, reducing appetite.
  » **5-HTP (5-hydroxytryptophan)**, a precursor to serotonin, can help reduce cravings and improve mood, impacting hunger signals from the hypothalamus.

2. **Pituitary Gland (Low Growth Hormone)**
   - **Get enough sleep:** Deep sleep promotes growth hormone secretion. Aim for seven to nine hours of quality sleep each night to support the pituitary's ability to release adequate growth hormone.
   - **Intermittent fasting:** Fasting has been shown to boost growth hormone levels naturally. Consider time-restricted eating to allow the pituitary gland to produce growth hormone without interference from constant insulin spikes.
   - **Exercise regularly:** High-intensity interval training (HIIT) and resistance training stimulate growth hormone production, which supports muscle growth and fat loss.
   - **Go dairy-free:** Recombinant bovine growth hormone (rBGH) is a synthetic (man-made) hormone that is marketed to dairy farmers to increase milk production in cows. It has been used in the United States since it was approved by the Food and Drug Administration (FDA) in 1993. Milk from cows given rBGH has higher levels of IGF-1, a hormone that normally helps some types of cells to grow. Several studies have found that IGF-1 levels at the high end of the normal range may influence the development of certain tumors.

- **Herbs and Supplements**
  » **Ashwagandha**, known as an adaptogen, supports overall hormone balance and can enhance sleep quality, which is essential for growth hormone production.
  » **L-arginine** is an amino acid that can stimulate growth hormone release, especially when taken before exercise.

3. **Thyroid Gland (Thyroid Dysfunction)**
   - **Increase iodine intake:** The thyroid requires iodine for hormone production. Incorporate iodine-rich foods like seaweed, iodized salt, and fish to support thyroid function.
   - **Avoid goitrogens:** Goitrogens (found in raw cruciferous vegetables like cabbage and broccoli) can interfere with thyroid function. Cooking these vegetables reduces their goitrogenic effect.
   - **Reduce exposure to fluoride and bromine:** These chemicals compete with iodine uptake in the thyroid. Use fluoride-free toothpaste, drink filtered water, and avoid bromine-rich processed foods to support thyroid health.
   - Avoid gluten.
   - **Herbs and Supplements**
     » **Iodine** is essential for thyroid hormone production. It is preferrable to get this predominantly from your diet. However, if you have been found to have low iodine levels, you could consider adding iodine-rich supplements.
     » **Selenium** is found in Brazil nuts. Just two each day can supply your daily selenium requirement. It is available as a supplement. It supports thyroid health and helps prevent thyroid hormone conversion issues.
     » **Bladder wrack** is a type of seaweed high in iodine that supports thyroid function.

4. **Gut Health (Low GLP-1 Levels)**
   - By now, most of us have heard of the popular weight loss medications Ozempic, Wegovy and Zepbound. These are GLP-1 agonists or stimulants that help suppress appetite for effective weight loss. However, there are ways to boost your GLP-1 levels naturally. This may take longer for an effect, but without the side effects.
   - **Increase fiber intake:** Dietary fiber promotes the release of GLP-1, a hormone that helps regulate blood sugar and reduces appetite. Fiber supplements like psyllium husk or oat bran can increase the excretion of fatty toxins in the stool. Aim for a diet rich in whole grains like quinoa, vegetables, and legumes. An increased intake of ground flaxseeds has been shown to increase butyrate, which in turn, can increase the body's production of GLP-1. This results in reduced appetite and an increase in fat-burning capabilities.
   - Drink bone broth or add collagen to food or drinks to help with a leaky gut.
   - **Eat probiotic-rich and fermented foods:** Foods like yogurt, kefir, sauerkraut, and kimchi promote a healthy gut microbiome, which plays a crucial role in the release of GLP-1.
   - **Limit processed foods, refined carbohydrates, preservatives, food colorings, and artificial ingredients:** These can harm gut bacteria, reducing the production of GLP-1. Focus on a diet with whole, unprocessed foods to support gut health and natural GLP-1 levels.
   - Increase the use of healthy fats like avocado oil and extra-virgin olive oil.
   - Drinking ginger tea has been shown to help block the reabsorption of fats and fatty toxins in the intestines.

- Adding a cup of oolong tea while eating a high-fat meal has been shown to increase the excretion of fats into the stool.
- **Herbs and Supplements**
    » **Probiotic supplements** contain beneficial bacteria that support gut health and improve GLP-1 production.
    » **Berberine** is an herbal extract that can modulate the gut microbiome and has been shown to increase GLP-1 levels.
    » **Slippery elm, licorice root, and marshmallow root** are soluble fibers that have been shown to soothe the gut lining, feed a healthy microbiome, and boost GLP-1 levels.
    » **Resveratrol** activates specific receptors in the intestinal lining, which then stimulates the production and secretion of GLP-1 from the intestinal L cells.
    » **Cinnamon** indirectly impacts GLP-1 release by potentially influencing the way glucose levels are absorbed in the intestines, leading to delayed gastric emptying.
    » **Turmeric** contains an active compound called curcumin which activates signaling pathways to increase GLP-1 secretion.
    » **L-glutamine** elevates intracellular cAMP (cyclic adenosine monophosphate), a second messenger molecule that plays a role in regulating biological processes like hormone action, energy metabolism, cell growth, and immune response. It has been shown to trigger the pathway responsible for GLP-1 secretion.
    » **Digestive enzymes**, when taken before each meal, help break down nutrients more efficiently.

5. **Stomach (High Ghrelin Levels)**
   - **Eat protein-rich meals:** Protein has been shown to reduce ghrelin levels, helping to keep hunger in check. Include lean proteins like chicken, fish, legumes, and eggs in your meals.
   - **Stay hydrated:** Drinking water before meals can help reduce ghrelin levels and control hunger. Aim for at least eight glasses of water per day.
   - **Manage stress:** Chronic stress increases ghrelin production, promoting hunger. Practice stress-relieving techniques like meditation, deep breathing exercises, or yoga.
   - Avoid snacking in between meals.
   - **Herbs and Supplements**
     » **Ginger** is known to help stabilize blood sugar levels and may reduce ghrelin levels, curbing appetite.
     » **Chromium picolinate** is a mineral that can help reduce food cravings and regulate hunger hormones.

6. **Liver (Decreased Metabolism)**
   - **Reduce alcohol consumption:** Alcohol impairs liver function, leading to a slower metabolism. Limit alcohol intake to support healthy liver function.
   - **Eat liver-friendly foods:** Foods like leafy greens, beets, and citrus fruits contain antioxidants that help detoxify the liver and improve metabolic rate.
   - **Herbs and Supplements**
     » **Milk thistle**, known for its liver-supporting properties, helps detoxify the liver and supports metabolism.
     » **Dandelion root** promotes liver health by improving bile production and aiding in toxin elimination.
     » **N-acetyl cysteine (NAC)** is a powerful antioxidant that supports liver detoxification processes.

- » **Turmeric** improves liver function and aids in the metabolic process.
- » **Glutathione** acts as a powerful antioxidant and is primarily responsible for detoxification processes within the liver cells, protecting it from damage caused by toxins and oxidative stress.

7. **Pancreas (Insulin Resistance)**
   - **Avoid artificial sweeteners, and limit sugar and refined carbs:** High sugar and carb intake can lead to insulin resistance and increased fat deposition. They can also disrupt gut health by disrupting the normal gut microbiome and increasing inflammation, which leads to fat depositing into the muscles and organs. They can also stimulate an increase in absorption of sugar in the intestines. So, even though they are advertised as "sugar substitutes," they can actually backfire and cause higher bloodsugars and disease. It contradicts what we think about sweeteners but they actually make it harder to clear sugar from the bloodstream. Furthermore, as artificial sweeteners lead to insulin resistance, this can cause excessive hunger and weight gain. Choose whole grains, fruits, and vegetables over refined options to improve insulin sensitivity.
   - **Incorporate cinnamon:** Cinnamon has been shown to improve insulin sensitivity. Add it to meals or beverages to help regulate blood sugar.
   - **Get regular physical activity:** Exercise helps cells become more responsive to insulin, lowering blood sugar levels and improving insulin sensitivity.

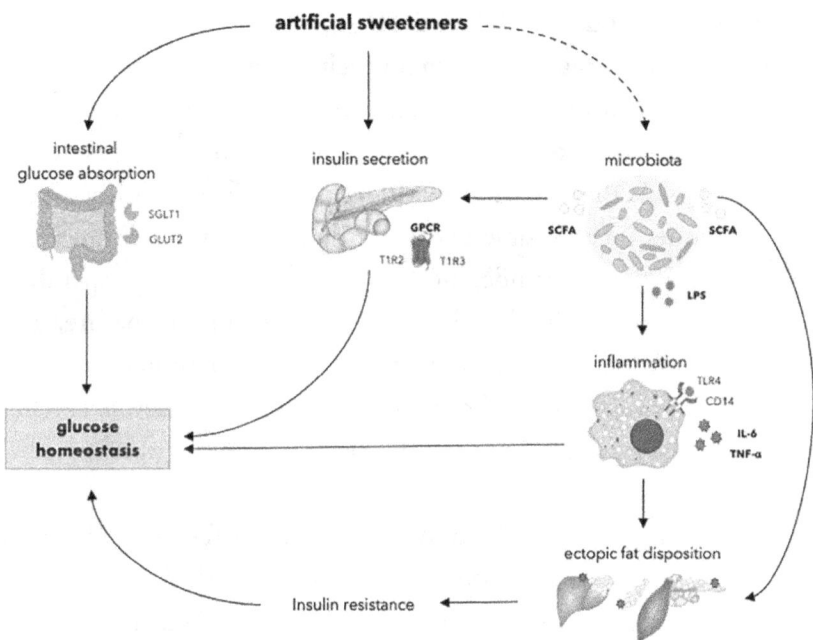

This Photo by Unknown Author is licensed under CC BY

- **Add chia seeds:** Due to their high fiber content, they can slow the absorption of sugar in the blood.
- **Drink apple cider vinegar:** Apple cider vinegar has been shown to improve blood sugar levels by delaying gastric emptying and increasing glucose uptake by cells. Drink two to three ounces of water with one tablespoon of apple cider vinegar before each meal.
- **Herbs and Supplements**
  » **Berberine**, known for its blood sugar-regulating effects, has been shown to improve insulin sensitivity.
  » **Cinnamon extract** supports insulin sensitivity and lowers blood sugar levels.
  » **Alpha-lipoic acid (ALA)** is an antioxidant that can help improve insulin sensitivity and reduce oxidative stress.

8. **Adrenal Glands (High Cortisol)**
   - **Practice stress management techniques:** High cortisol from chronic stress promotes fat storage. Incorporate relaxation techniques like mindfulness, meditation, breathing exercises, massage therapy, or yoga to lower cortisol levels. Other techniques include slow and low-impact exercises, affirmations, practicing gratitude, smiling, dancing, laughing, spending more time with loved ones, spending time in nature, and limiting screen time on your phone and computer.
   - **Limit caffeine intake:** Excessive caffeine can elevate cortisol levels, especially in stressful situations. Instead, opt for herbal teas or water.
   - **Eat magnesium-rich and nutrient-dense foods:** Magnesium can help reduce cortisol production. Include leafy greens, nuts, avocados, seeds, and whole grains in your diet. Adopting an anti-inflammatory diet high in omega-3 fatty acids (such as fatty fish, chia seeds, and flaxseeds) has been proven to have the most benefits.
   - Limit alcohol intake.
   - Drink coconut water with a dash of Celtic salt and lime juice.
   - **Herbs and Supplements**
     » **Rhodiola rosea** is an adaptogen that helps reduce cortisol levels and combats stress-induced fatigue.
     » **Holy basil (tulsi)** is a revered plant in the traditional Indian medicine system, Ayurveda. It is known for its benefits in lowering blood sugars, antioxidant properties, and reducing anxiety. Known for its cortisol-lowering effects, Holy basil supports adrenal health and reduces stress.

- » **Magnesium** helps relax muscles and reduces cortisol levels, especially when taken before bed.
- » **Ashwagandha** is another adaptogen that may help calm the brain, lower blood pressure, and improve the immune system.
- » **Lemon balm**, a plant in the mint family, has been shown to reduce stress and anxiety, improve sleep, and help with digestive issues.
- » **Vitamin D**, when present in lower levels, has been associated with higher cortisol levels. Supplementation with vitamin D stimulates the vitamin D receptors in the hypothalamus, which in turn regulates the adrenal gland's production of cortisol.

9. **Reproductive Organs (Excess Estrogen)**
   - **Limit exposure to xenoestrogens:** Xenoestrogens are synthetic compounds that mimic estrogen and can be found in plastics, cosmetics, and pesticides. Use glass or stainless-steel containers, and choose organic and natural personal care products, to reduce exposure.
   - **Eat cruciferous vegetables:** Vegetables like broccoli, cauliflower, and kale contain compounds that help the liver process and excrete excess estrogen.
   - **Increase fiber intake:** Fiber helps bind and remove excess estrogen through the digestive tract. Aim for twenty-five to thirty grams of fiber per day from foods like fruits, vegetables, and whole grains.
   - **Increase foods that balance estrogen:** This includes raw carrots, citrus fruits, lentils, grass-fed butter, eggs, Brazil nuts, ground flaxseeds, and green tea. Avoid excess meat intake, especially non-grass-fed meats. Avoid GMO foods.

- **Herbs and Supplements**
  - » **Diindolylmethane (DIM)** is a compound derived from cruciferous vegetables that helps metabolize excess estrogen.
  - » **Vitex (chasteberry)** supports hormone balance by modulating prolactin levels, which can influence estrogen balance.
  - » **Calcium-D-glucarate** assists in the detoxification of excess estrogen in the liver, helping to clear it from the body.

10. Fat Cells (Leptin Resistance)
    - **Consume omega-3 fatty acids:** Omega-3s can improve leptin sensitivity. Sources include fatty fish (such as salmon), chia seeds, and walnuts.
    - **Eat more high-chlorophyll foods:** Incorporating seaweed, algae, and foods high in chlorophyll has been shown to decrease fat absorption and increase disposal of fat-soluble toxins. Foods high in chlorophyll include spinach, broccoli, cabbage, asparagus, brussels sprouts, kale, parsley, and other green, leafy vegetables.
    - **Avoid processed foods:** High-calorie, processed foods can lead to leptin resistance. Focus on whole foods to help the body respond better to leptin's signals.
    - **Avoid high-fructose corn syrup** and excess sweet fruits which have too much fructose.
    - **Incorporate regular exercise:** Physical activity has been shown to improve leptin sensitivity, helping regulate appetite and reduce food cravings. When done on a regular basis, studies have confirmed the reversal of fatty liver disease.
    - Avoid sleep deprivation which can increase leptin.

- Use of an infrared sauna can promote sweating out toxins from the skin and fat cells.
- **Herbs and Supplements**
  - **Fish oil (omega-3 fatty acids)** improve leptin sensitivity and help reduce inflammation in fat cells.
  - **Turmeric (curcumin)** contains anti-inflammatory properties that may improve leptin sensitivity.
  - **Resveratrol**, found in red wine and available as a supplement, can help combat leptin resistance.

Conclusion

By focusing on natural approaches to address each of these pathways, you can reduce the impact of obesogens on your body. These lifestyle changes not only target weight management but also promote better overall health by supporting hormonal balance, enhancing metabolism, and reducing chronic inflammation. With a consistent, holistic approach, you can significantly lower your exposure to obesogens and improve your body's ability to maintain a healthy weight naturally.

CHAPTER FOURTEEN:

No More Plastics! Reducing Plastic Use to Minimize Exposure to EDCs in Everyday Life

BPA and Phthalates: Silent Culprits

BPA and phthalates, commonly found in various plastic items, have been associated with numerous health issues due to their ability to mimic or interfere with the body's hormones. Because they can trigger obesity and impact fertility, it's vital to recognize their sneaky entry into our bodies via everyday products and take preventive actions.

Plastic Leaching: An Unseen Hazard

When plastics are exposed to certain conditions like heat and acidity, the risk of leaching, whereby chemicals transfer from the plastic into the contained food or beverage, increases.

- **Heat exposure:** Microwaving plastic containers or leaving them in a hot environment (like in a car) can facilitate the migration of harmful EDCs into the contained food.

- **Acid interaction:** Acidic foods and beverages, like tomato sauce or lemon juice, can magnify the leaching of chemicals from plastic containers.
- **Oils and fatty foods:** EDCs are fat soluble, and so are attracted to high-fat foods like ghee, coconut oil, and dairy products.

Reducing Plastic and Reducing Harm
Be a Conscious Consumer
- **Choose glass and metal:** Whenever possible, opt for glass, stainless steel, or other alternatives for storage containers, water bottles, and straws.
- **Avoid single-use plastics:** Resist the convenience of single-use plastics by adopting reusable items like bags, cups, and cutlery.

Get Acquainted with Recycling Codes
- **Understand symbols:** Learn to recognize and understand the recycling symbols on plastic items to avoid those known to leach harmful chemicals. For example, the #3 symbol indicates the presence of phthalates.

Be Mindful of Your Grocery Shopping List
- **Choose fresh over packaged:** Purchase fresh produce instead of those wrapped in plastic.
- **Don't purchase acidic foods in plastic:** Look for foods stored in glass containers.
- **Buy in bulk:** Choose bulk buying options using your own reusable containers to diminish consumption of plastic packaging.

Advocate for Plastic Reduction
Community Initiatives
- **Organize cleanups:** Establish or participate in local cleanup events to remove plastic waste from natural environments.

- **Support plastic-free establishments:** Encourage and frequent businesses that are committed to reducing plastic usage.

Be a Voice for Change
- **Advocate for policies:** Lend your voice and support to policies that aim to reduce plastic production and use at local, national, and global levels.
- **Educate others:** Raise awareness about the dangers of EDCs in plastics, and inspire others to join the movement toward reduction and safer alternatives.

Embrace a Plastic-Free Life

Begin at Home
- **Survey your plastic use:** Identify alternatives for plastic items used in your home, especially in the kitchen, bathroom, and laundry room.
- **Avoid heating food in foam or plastic:** Incorporate tips and habits to avoid plastic leaching into your daily life, such as utilizing glass or ceramic for storing and microwaving foods, especially those that are acidic or require heating.

Empower Through Education
- **Inform and inspire:** Use your journey as a tool to educate and inspire others to embark on a similar path, amplifying the impact and extending the reach of plastic reduction efforts.

Future Innovations and Alternatives in Plastic

Bioplastics and Beyond
- **Explore alternatives:** Search for new options like bioplastics and other innovative materials that promise reduced environmental and health impacts.

Technology and Recycling
- **Enhanced recycling:** Explore advancements in recycling technology that may offer more robust solutions for plastic waste management.

Navigating through the ubiquitous presence of plastics requires a dedicated effort and a combination of personal choices, community actions, and advocacy. Remember to start small, and know that every new, small action or change contributes to a larger impact long-term. If you are familiar with the *Avengers* movies, "We are in the end game!"

CHAPTER FIFTEEN:

A Breath of Fresh Air: How to Reduce Indoor and Outdoor Pollutants

Living in a modern society, we are perpetually surrounded by a myriad of chemicals that pervade our environment. Indoors, pollutants lurk in the air we breathe, the furniture we use, and the cleaning products we choose. Outdoors, vehicular emissions, pesticides, and industrial pollutants are omnipresent, complicating our efforts to maintain a clean and healthy environment. Among these pollutants, endocrine-disrupting chemicals (EDCs) are particularly insidious, subtly interfering with our hormonal systems and precipitating adverse health effects. Armed with knowledge and effective strategies, we can mitigate our exposure to these disruptive forces, cultivating an environment that supports rather than hinders our well-being.

Our homes, often regarded as safe havens, can sometimes be the source of substances that harm our well-being. Indoor pollutants, prevalent yet overlooked, play subtle roles in affecting our health, particularly in relation to the endocrine system. The array of pollutants is vast, ranging from the delightful scent of incense to the fresh spritz of air fresheners. Let's delve into understanding how seemingly benign household items can be hidden conduits for endocrine-disrupting chemicals (EDCs).

- **Incense:** Incense, known for its spiritual and aromatic significance, is a common indoor pollutant. When burned, it releases particulate matter, volatile organic compounds (VOCs), and other harmful substances into the air. These pollutants, though veiled in fragrant smoke, can adversely impact indoor air quality and may have potential effects on endocrine function.
- **Air fresheners:** Air fresheners, while effective in masking odors, often contain phthalates and other chemicals that can act as EDCs. Their continuous use can lead to a buildup of these substances in the indoor environment, contributing to an increased risk of endocrine disruption.
- **Candles:** Candles, especially those made from paraffin wax, can emit VOCs, including formaldehyde and benzene, when burned. Opting for candles made from beeswax or soy can be a healthier alternative.
- **Cleaning products:** As highlighted before, cleaning products may be filled with chemicals that can be endocrine disruptors. It is essential to choose products with the least harmful ingredients, ensuring a cleaner and safer indoor environment.
- **Cosmetics and personal care products:** Items like deodorants, lotions, and shampoos often have chemicals that can act as EDCs. These substances can be absorbed through the skin or inhaled, thereby finding pathways into our bodies.

Indoor Air Improvement Strategies

- **Ventilate:** Regularly ventilate your indoor spaces. Fresh air helps dissipate the concentration of indoor pollutants, including volatile organic compounds (VOCs), facilitating a healthier breathing environment.
- **Reduce volatile organic compounds (VOCs):** VOCs are a group of carbon-based chemicals that easily evaporate at room temperature. Common sources include household cleaning agents, paint, and even some cosmetics. VOCs are notorious for their contribution to indoor air pollution. Being informed about and choosing products with lower VOC content can substantially reduce indoor pollution levels.
- **Choose furniture wisely:** Many furniture pieces contain chemicals like flame retardants that can off-gas over time and may be harmful. Selecting furniture that is certified as low in VOCs and that doesn't contain polybrominated diphenyl ethers (PBDEs) is advisable.
- **Be mindful when selecting cleaning products:** Choose cleaning products that are labeled as eco-friendly or are made from natural ingredients. These typically have fewer harmful chemicals and lower VOC content. Be wary of products with strong fragrances, as they often contain phthalates.
- **Minimize dust:** Regular cleaning practices such as dusting and vacuuming can help in reducing the accumulation of pollutants that settle in household dust.

Outdoor Air Exposure Strategies

- **Stay informed about air quality:** Make it a habit to check the air quality index in your locality. On days when pollution levels are high, consider staying indoors or avoiding strenuous outdoor activities.

- **Cultivate green spaces:** Having plants in and around your living spaces can help in improving air quality. Plants can absorb a multitude of pollutants, acting as natural air purifiers.
- **Choose your outdoor activities wisely:** When engaging in outdoor physical activities, opt for areas that are away from heavy traffic and industrial emissions to reduce your exposure to pollutants.
- **Use masks and respirators:** In highly polluted environments, consider the use of masks or respirators which can help in reducing the inhalation of harmful particles.

Conclusion

Awareness is a powerful tool. Understanding the potential sources of indoor pollutants allows for informed choices, minimizing exposure to substances that might disrupt the delicate balance of your endocrine system. Crafting a mindful living space, free from harmful pollutants, can be an incremental step toward fostering health and well-being amid a backdrop of evolving environmental challenges.

While complete avoidance of EDCs in the environment might be a daunting task, strategic actions can substantially mitigate their impact. Cultivating awareness, making informed choices, and adopting practical measures are crucial in navigating the labyrinth of pollutants that characterize our modern landscapes. In this journey of mitigation, each step counts, collectively weaving the fabric of a resilient and health-supporting environment.

CHAPTER SIXTEEN:

Spring Cleaning Anytime: Using Safe Household Products and Eliminating EDC-Laden Products

In the pursuit of maintaining a clean and healthy home, we often overlook how some commonly used household products may be counterproductive to our well-being. Many of these products contain endocrine-disrupting chemicals (EDCs) that can subtly impact on our health. Many release volatile organic compounds that enter the body through inhalation, which evades the first pass of metabolism in the liver. Most products do not list all of their chemicals, and nearly all contain phthalates, ethanolamine, and toluene. Recognizing and eliminating these products is essential in creating a safer home environment.

Identifying EDC-Laden Products in Your Home

Understanding the sources of EDCs in household products is the first step toward making safer choices.

- **Cleaning agents:** Many conventional cleaning products contain EDCs like phthalates (often hidden under the term "fragrance") and triclosan. Bleach can release carbon tetrachloride which contributes to greenhouse gases, depletes the body of glutathione, and is toxic to the liver and kidneys. Degreasing agents, oven cleansers, and glass cleaners can cause liver and kidney damage and fertility difficulties. These chemicals can disrupt hormonal balance and have been linked to various health issues.
- **Air fresheners and scented candles:** Products designed to make our homes smell pleasant, such as air fresheners and scented candles, often contain synthetic fragrances that can release phthalates and other EDCs into the air.
- **Nonstick cookware:** Pans and pots coated with nonstick surfaces are often made using chemicals like perfluorooctanoic acid (PFOA) which have been associated with endocrine disruption.
- **Plastic containers and food packaging:** Many plastics, including food packaging and storage containers, can contain BPA or phthalates, especially when these plastics are old, damaged, or heated.
- **Personal care products:** Items like shampoos, soaps, lotions, and deodorants can contain parabens, phthalates, and other chemicals that act as EDCs.
- **Laundry detergents:** Some detergents contain ingredients that can disrupt hormonal function, including phthalates (for fragrance) and other chemicals.

Safe Alternatives for Household Cleaning

Switching to safer alternatives can significantly reduce your exposure to EDCs.

- **Natural cleaning solutions:** Employ natural cleaning agents like vinegar, baking soda, and lemon juice. These alternatives are effective for many cleaning tasks without the risks associated with synthetic chemicals.
- **Eco-friendly commercial products:** Choose cleaning products certified as environmentally-friendly and free from harmful chemicals.

Detoxifying Kitchen Practices

- **Food storage:** Transition from plastic containers to glass or stainless steel to avoid the leaching of chemicals.
- **Cookware choices:** Choose safer cookware options like cast iron, stainless steel, or ceramic.

Revamping Laundry Practices

- **Natural laundry detergents:** Buy detergents that are free from harsh chemicals and synthetic fragrances.
- **Fabric softener alternatives:** Use wool dryer balls instead of conventional fabric softeners or dryer sheets.

Personal Care Product Reform

- **Safer personal care products:** Choose products with natural ingredients and those that are free from harmful additives like parabens and phthalates.
- **DIY products:** Consider making your own personal care products using simple, natural ingredients.

Conclusion

Conducting a thorough spring cleaning of your household products is not just about cleanliness; it's about safeguarding your health from hidden chemical threats. By identifying and replacing products laden with EDCs, you can create a safer and healthier home environment. This ongoing journey toward a toxin-free home requires vigilance but is a necessary step in fostering a holistic and health-conscious lifestyle.

CHAPTER SEVENTEEN:

Self-Care for Your Body: Choosing Clean Personal Care Products

In our daily self-care routines, we often use a variety of personal care products, from cosmetics and sunscreens to shampoos, lotions, deodorants, nail polish, and hair dyes. While these products help us look and feel our best, many contain a cocktail of endocrine-disrupting chemicals (EDCs) that can have long-term health implications and impact out hormonal health. This chapter is dedicated to understanding these risks and offers guidance on making safer choices.

Understanding EDCs in Personal Care Products

- **Parabens:** Commonly used as preservatives in a wide range of cosmetics and skincare products, parabens can mimic estrogen and disrupt hormonal balance.
- **Phthalates:** Often found in fragranced products like lotions and perfumes, phthalates are known for their potential endocrine-disrupting effects.

- **Triclosan:** Used in antibacterial soaps and some toothpastes, triclosan can interfere with thyroid function and other hormonal processes.
- **Sulfates:** Common in shampoos and body washes, sulfates can strip away natural oils and may be contaminated with dioxane, a suspected carcinogen.

EDCs in Common Personal Care Products

- **Cosmetics:** Many makeup products, including foundations, lipsticks, and eyeliners, may contain EDCs like parabens and phthalates. These chemicals can be absorbed through the skin, potentially disrupting hormonal balance.
- **Sunscreens:** Chemical sunscreens often contain ingredients like oxybenzone and octinoxate, known to have endocrine-disrupting effects. They can mimic hormones and cause skin allergies.
- **Deodorants:** Some deodorants and antiperspirants include aluminum compounds, parabens, and triclosan, which can mimic estrogen and other hormones. Prolonged exposure to these substances might be linked to various health concerns.
- **Nail polish:** Many nail polishes contain dibutyl phthalate (DBP), toluene, and formaldehyde—known as the "toxic trio." These chemicals can disrupt endocrine functions and pose other health risks.
- **Hair dyes:** Permanent and semipermanent hair dyes often contain ammonia, peroxide, p-phenylenediamine (PPD), and resorcinol, which can have hormone-disrupting effects and may cause skin irritation or allergies.

Choosing Safer Personal Care Products

- **Read labels carefully:** Become adept at reading and understanding product labels. Avoid products with known EDCs like parabens, phthalates, and triclosan.
- **Seek certified products:** Look for certifications like USDA organic, EWG verified, or similar, which often indicate a product is free from many harmful chemicals.
- **Fragrance-free options:** Choose fragrance-free products or those scented with natural essential oils instead of synthetic fragrances.
- **Natural and organic brands:** Support brands that are committed to producing clean and safe personal care products.

Choosing Safer Alternatives

- **Natural and organic makeup:** Purchase makeup that is made using natural or organic ingredients and is free from parabens, phthalates, and other harmful chemicals.
- **Mineral-based sunscreens:** Choose sunscreens with mineral-based ingredients like zinc oxide and titanium dioxide, which are less likely to contain harmful chemicals.
- **Aluminum-free deodorants:** Look for natural deodorants that use ingredients like baking soda, arrowroot powder, or mineral salts instead of aluminum and parabens.
- **Nontoxic nail polish:** Seek out nail polish brands that are "three-free" (free from DBP, toluene, and formaldehyde), or even "five-free" or "seven-free" for more comprehensive safety.
- **Natural hair dye alternatives:** Consider using natural hair dyes that use plant-based ingredients or henna. Be cautious even with natural dyes, and conduct patch tests for allergic reactions.

DIY Personal Care Products
- **Homemade alternatives:** Creating your own personal care products—such as deodorants, face masks, or scrubs—using natural ingredients can be a fun and safe way to reduce exposure to harmful chemicals.

Supporting Skin Health Naturally
- **Nutrient-rich diet:** A diet rich in antioxidants, vitamins, and minerals supports skin health, potentially reducing the need for numerous skincare products.
- **Gentle care:** Adopt gentle cleaning and exfoliating routines that maintain the skin's natural balance.

Making Informed Choices
- **Stay informed:** Keep abreast of the latest research and recommendations regarding safe personal care products.
- **Prioritize health over trends:** Choose products based on their safety profile rather than on popularity or trends.

Conclusion
Navigating the array of personal care products available can be daunting, especially when trying to avoid EDCs. By making informed choices, seeking safer alternatives, and even crafting your own products, you can significantly reduce your body's chemical burden. Adopting a cleaner, more natural approach to personal care is not only beneficial for our endocrine health but also aligns with a holistic view of wellness and environmental responsibility. Remember, the choices we make for our personal care have broader implications for our long-term health and the health of our planet.

CHAPTER EIGHTEEN:

Relax, Relate, and Release! Emphasizing Relaxation and Stress Management for Overall Well-Being

The interplay between stress, our body's physiological responses, and the impacts of endocrine-disrupting chemicals (EDCs) forms a complex web that influences our overall health. In this fast-paced world, stress has become an inevitable part of life, yet its management is crucial, especially when considering its interaction with EDCs. The long-term activation of the stress response system can lead to excess production of the stress hormone cortisol, which then disrupts many of the body's processes. This, in turn, can lead to weight gain, depression, anxiety, digestive issues, sleep abnormalities, high blood pressure, decreased memory, and an increased risk for heart attacks and strokes. This chapter explores the intricate relationship between stress, gut health, liver function, cortisol levels, and how EDCs can exacerbate stress responses in the body.

TOXIC OVERLOAD: The Invisible Endocrine-Disrupting Chemicals Making Us Sick, Fat, and Tired

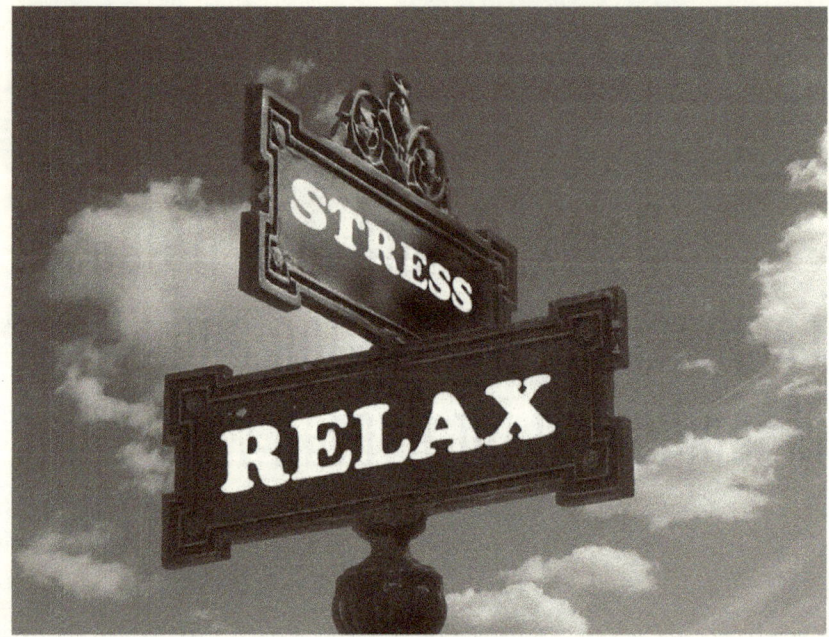

CC BY 4.0

Understanding the Stress Response

- **Cortisol and the adrenal glands:** In response to stress, our adrenal glands secrete cortisol, a hormone that helps regulate metabolism, immune response, and stress reaction. While cortisol is vital for survival, its chronic elevation can lead to health issues.
- **Impact on gut health:** Stress can alter the gut microbiota composition and increase intestinal permeability, often referred to as "leaky gut," which can exacerbate inflammation and lead to a host of health issues.
- **Effect on liver function:** Chronic stress can impair liver function, affecting its ability to detoxify the body, including the processing and elimination of EDCs.

The Interaction of EDCs and Stress Responses

- **Amplifying stress effects:** EDCs can exacerbate the effects of stress on the body. For instance, certain EDCs can affect the normal functioning of the adrenal glands, leading to dysregulated cortisol production.
- **Compromising detoxification under stress:** EDCs can further strain the liver's detoxification capacity, particularly when one is under stress, as the body's resources are redirected to immediate survival mechanisms rather than to detoxification processes.
- **Inflammation and microbiome disruption:** EDC-induced inflammation can alter the gut environment, making it more hostile for certain beneficial bacteria. This inflammation can stem from direct irritation of the gut lining or from systemic effects caused by EDC-induced immune responses.
- **Interaction with gut-brain axis:** The gut-brain axis, a bidirectional communication pathway, can be influenced by EDCs. For example, EDC-induced stress responses can affect gut motility and secretion, further impacting the gut microbiome and its functions.
- **Gut health and EDCs:** The combination of stress and exposure to EDCs can significantly impact gut health, exacerbating issues like dysbiosis and leaky gut, which can lead to systemic health problems.
- **Altering gut microbiota composition:** EDCs can directly impact the composition and diversity of the gut microbiota. These chemicals can create an environment that favors the growth of harmful bacteria over beneficial ones, leading to dysbiosis.
- **Impairing gut barrier function:** EDCs can weaken the intestinal barrier (increasing gut permeability), often referred

to as "leaky gut." This condition allows bacteria and toxins to "leak" into the bloodstream, causing inflammation and further disrupting gut microbiome balance.

Understanding Electromagnetic Fields (EMFs)

Electromagnetic fields (EMFs) are areas of energy that are produced by electronic devices, power lines, and wireless communication technologies. EMFs are categorized into low-frequency (nonionizing) and high-frequency (ionizing) radiation. Low-frequency EMFs, which include those emitted by cell phones, Wi-Fi routers, and computers, have been a growing concern due to their potential impact on health and well-being.

EMF Exposure and Its Impact on Melatonin Production

Melatonin is a hormone produced by the pineal gland that plays a critical role in regulating sleep-wake cycles, also known as our circadian rhythm, and promoting restful sleep. It is often referred to as the "sleep hormone" because of its direct influence on circadian rhythms. However, melatonin also has antioxidant properties and contributes to stress reduction and immune system support. It unfortunately decreases with age, which explains how insomnia worsens as we get older.

Research Highlights

1. **Suppression of Melatonin Production**
   » Studies have shown that exposure to EMFs, particularly at night, can suppress the production of melatonin. This is thought to occur because EMFs may interfere with the pineal gland's ability to release melatonin by disrupting the brain's perception of natural light and dark cycles (Burch et al. 1999).

- » EMFs from devices like smartphones and Wi-Fi routers can emit artificial blue light, which mimics daylight and signals the brain to stay alert, thereby inhibiting melatonin release (Höhn et al. 2024). Common sources of blue light come from TVs, computers, and cell phones.
- » Fluoride has been shown to interfere with pineal production of melatonin.
- » Stress, caffeine, alcohol, and excess cortisol have all been shown to suppress melatonin secretion.

2. **Sleep Quality and Circadian Rhythm Disruption**
   - » Reduced melatonin levels due to prolonged EMF exposure can lead to sleep disturbances, poor-quality sleep, and circadian rhythm disruptions. Insufficient melatonin can impair the body's ability to fall asleep and stay asleep, leading to an increased risk of stress, fatigue, and mood disorders (Halgamuge 2013). Low melatonin levels can inhibit our ability to enter the stage-four REM sleep needed for restorative effects.
   - » The next diagram shows the numerous downstream effects of sleep disruption. Poor sleep can have long-term effects on cortisol production, thyroid function, fat metabolism, gut health, and even glucose management. Regular exercise, proper diet, and an adequate sleep schedule can promote proper hormonal balance and metabolism.

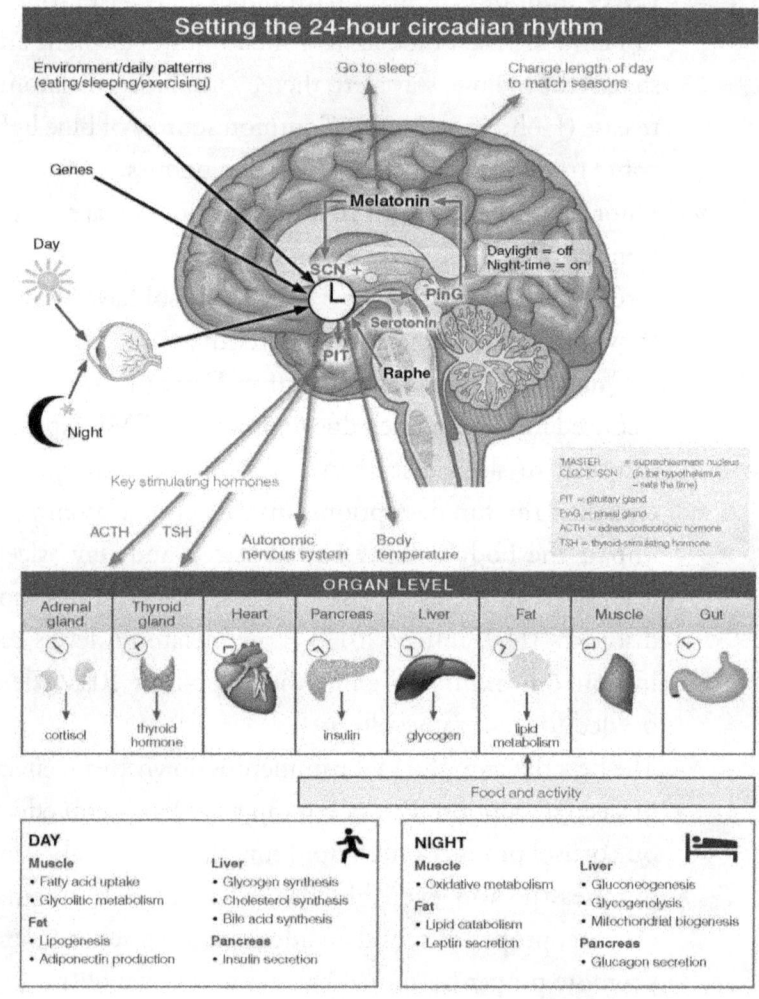

This Photo by Unknown Author is licensed under CC BY-SA

Implications for Stress and Well-Being
1. **Increased Stress Response**
   » Chronic exposure to EMFs has been linked to increased stress responses in the body. Lower levels of melatonin, which plays a role in stress management and antioxidant

defense, can lead to heightened stress, inflammation, and oxidative damage (Reiter et al. 2014).
   » Melatonin acts as a natural buffer against stress by modulating the hypothalamic-pituitary-adrenal (HPA) axis, the body's primary stress response system. Reduced melatonin can therefore lead to a heightened cortisol response, further exacerbating stress and its physiological effects (Hardeland 2008).
2. **Weakened Immune System**
   » Melatonin supports the immune system by reducing oxidative stress and promoting the activity of immune cells. EMF-induced reductions in melatonin levels can impair immune function, making the body more susceptible to illness and reducing its ability to manage chronic stress (Reiter et al. 2014).

Tips for Reducing EMF Exposure and Supporting Melatonin Levels

1. **Limit Screen Time Before Bed**
   » Avoid using electronic devices like smartphones, tablets, and computers at least an hour before bedtime. If screen use is unavoidable, consider using blue light-blocking glasses or apps that reduce blue light exposure to support natural melatonin production.
2. **Create an EMF-Free Sleep Environment**
   » Keep electronic devices out of the bedroom or place them in airplane mode while sleeping. Consider unplugging Wi-Fi routers at night and using wired connections instead of wireless, when possible.
   » Put cell phones in airplane mode to reduce EMF emissions at bedtime.

- Avoid using electric blankets or heating pads at night.
- Use a blue light filter on your computer and cell phone.
- Wear blue light-blocking glasses at sundown to reduce effects while watching TV or while browsing the internet.
- Use EMF protection earbuds with a microphone and adapter instead of placing your cell phone directly on your ears.

3. **Incorporate Melatonin-Boosting Practices**
   - **Exposure to natural light:** Spend time outdoors during the day to reinforce your body's natural circadian rhythm.
   - **Early bedtime:** Set a steady and stable time for sleep, ideally between 10:00 and 11:00 p.m.
   - Reduce all light sources in the room during sleep.
   - **Room temperature:** Try to set the room temperature close to seventy degrees during sleep.
   - **Supplementation:** Melatonin supplements can be considered as a short-term solution to improve sleep quality and manage jet lag or stress-related sleep disturbances. However, it is essential to consult with a health-care provider before using melatonin supplements. Long-term use may suppress natural secretion of melatonin. Taking one to two grams of glycine at bedtime can boost serotonin and melatonin.
   - **Dietary sources:** Include foods that promote melatonin production, such as cherries, bananas, oats, and walnuts, which naturally contain melatonin or its precursor, tryptophan.

4. **Grounding Techniques**
   - **Earthing or grounding:** This practice involves direct skin contact with the earth (e.g., walking barefoot on grass or sand). Some studies suggest that grounding can help

neutralize free radicals and reduce the impact of EMFs on the body, potentially supporting melatonin production (Chevalier et al. 2012).

Herbs and Supplements to Support Relaxation and Melatonin Production

- **Herbal teas:** Chamomile, valerian root, and passionflower teas can promote relaxation and improve sleep quality.
- **Magnesium:** A supplement known for its calming properties, magnesium can help reduce stress and support melatonin production.
- **L-tryptophan and 5-HTP:** These are supplements that act as precursors to serotonin and melatonin to help regulate sleep and mood.

Strategies for Managing Stress

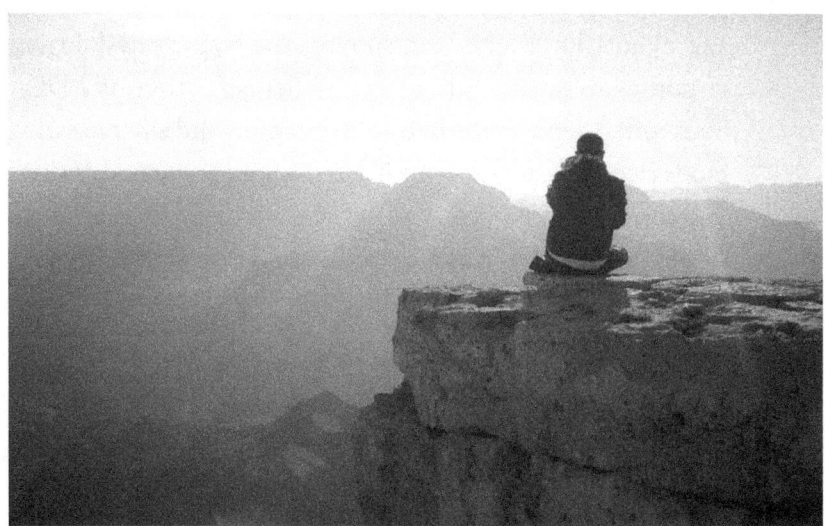

This Photo by Unknown Author is licensed under CC BY-SA

- **Mindfulness and relaxation techniques:** Practices such as meditation, yoga, massage, and deep breathing exercises can significantly reduce stress levels, helping to regulate cortisol production.
- **Keep a journal:** Writing down racing thoughts and making daily notes of gratitude have been shown to reduce stress and improve sleep.
- **Regular physical activity:** Engaging in regular exercise can alleviate stress and improve the body's resilience to both stress and the harmful effects of EDCs.
- **Adequate sleep:** Ensuring sufficient quality sleep is vital in managing stress and supporting the body's detoxification processes.
- **Use hobbies:** Find ways to use music, reading, painting, dancing, humor, movie watching, or spending time with family and friends.
- **Nutritional support:** A balanced diet, rich in antioxidants and essential nutrients, can support the body's physiological responses to stress and aid in the detoxification of EDCs. Stress often depletes the body of B vitamins and zinc, so eating foods rich in these nutrients helps to support the body's stress response.
- **Avoid unhealthy ways to reduce stress:** Limit alcohol, tobacco, drugs, and fast foods.

Conclusion

Understanding and managing stress is not just about enhancing our mental well-being; it's also a crucial aspect of maintaining our physical health, especially in relation to the impacts of EDCs. By adopting comprehensive strategies for stress management, we can support our body's resilience against the multifaceted challenges posed by stress and

EDCs. This holistic approach to relaxation, stress management, and self-care is a key component in our journey toward overall well-being and long-term health.

CHAPTER NINETEEN:

Implementing the Battle on a Budget: Cost-Effective Approaches to Reducing EDC Exposures

Combating exposure to endocrine-disrupting chemicals (EDCs) is a necessary pursuit for maintaining good health, but it can often seem financially daunting. The good news is that reducing EDC exposure doesn't have to break the bank. This chapter explores cost-effective approaches and practical tips for minimizing EDCs in everyday life, ensuring that these strategies are accessible and sustainable for everyone, regardless of budget.

Cost-Effective Approaches to Reducing EDC Exposures
1. **Prioritize Your Purchases**
    » Focus first on replacing items that you use frequently or that have high EDC risks. For instance, switching to a glass water bottle instead of plastic is a simple, one-time investment with long-term benefits.

2. **DIY Cleaning and Personal Care Products**
   » Homemade cleaning solutions using vinegar, baking soda, and lemon can be cheaper and just as effective as store-bought products. Similarly, creating your own personal care items like deodorants or scrubs from natural ingredients can be cost-effective and EDC-free.
3. **Buy in Bulk**
   » Purchasing whole foods in bulk can be cheaper and will reduce exposure to EDCs often found in the packaging of processed foods.
4. **Choose Local and Seasonal Produce**
   » Buying local and in-season fruits and vegetables can be more affordable, and these are less likely to be heavily treated with pesticides, compared to out-of-season or imported produce.

Practical Tips for Incorporating Strategies into Daily Life

1. **Educate Yourself and Others**
   » Knowledge is power, and it's free. Learn about EDCs, and share information with friends and family to make informed decisions together.
2. **Be Resourceful with What You Have**
   » Before purchasing new items, assess what you already own that can serve a similar purpose. For example, glass jars from food can be repurposed for storage.
3. **Gradual Transition**
   » Don't feel pressured to make all the changes at once. Gradually replacing products as they run out is less overwhelming and more budget-friendly.

4. **Use Technology Wisely**
    » Utilize apps and websites that offer information on the safest products and those with the least environmental impact. Many of these resources are free and can guide your shopping choices.
5. **Invest in Reusables**
    » Items like cloth shopping bags, reusable silicone baking sheets, or beeswax wraps may have an initial cost but will save you money in the long term as they replace disposable, often plastic, items.
6. **Minimize and Simplify**
    » Reducing overall consumption not only saves money but also limits potential EDC exposure. Simplifying your lifestyle to what is essential can have profound health and financial benefits.

Conclusion

Engaging in the battle against EDCs on a budget is entirely feasible and can even lead to a more mindful and sustainable lifestyle. By prioritizing, being resourceful, and adopting a step-by-step approach, you can effectively reduce your exposure to harmful chemicals without overextending your financial resources. This journey, when approached thoughtfully, can not only enhance your personal health but also contribute positively to environmental conservation.

PART THREE:

Winning the War! Exploring Alternative Approaches to Reach Your Goal

CHAPTER TWENTY:

Chinese Medicine Perspective on Combating EDC Effects

Traditional Chinese medicine (TCM) offers a holistic and integrative approach to health, emphasizing the balance and harmony of the body's internal systems. In the context of combating the effects of endocrine-disrupting chemicals (EDCs), TCM provides a unique perspective, focusing on strengthening the body's natural defenses and restoring balance. This chapter delves into the principles of TCM and how they can be applied to mitigate the impacts of EDCs.

Fundamental Concepts of TCM in Detoxification
1. **Qi (Energy) and Blood Circulation**
    - » TCM emphasizes the importance of maintaining smooth flow of qi and blood throughout the body. Techniques such as acupuncture, tai chi, and qigong are believed to enhance circulation and promote detoxification.

2. **Yin-Yang Balance**
   » EDCs can disrupt the delicate balance of yin (nourishing, cooling energy) and yang (active, warming energy) in the body. TCM seeks to restore this balance through dietary recommendations, herbal remedies, and lifestyle adjustments.
3. **Strengthening the Liver Function**
   » In TCM, the liver is crucial for detoxification and maintaining the free flow of qi. Herbs that support liver health and detoxifying functions are often recommended.

TCM Practices for Combating EDCs
1. **Acupuncture**
   » Used to stimulate specific points in the body to improve qi flow, reduce stress, and enhance overall well-being, acupuncture can be crucial in the body's response to EDCs.
2. **Herbal Medicine**
   » TCM prescribes a variety of herbs that are believed to detoxify the body and support organ systems, such as the liver and kidneys, impacted by EDCs.
3. **Dietary Therapy**
   » TCM promotes a balanced diet with a focus on whole, unprocessed foods. Foods that are believed to support detoxification include green, leafy vegetables, berries, and teas like green tea and dandelion tea.
4. **Mind-Body Practices**
   » Techniques such as tai chi and qigong are not only physical exercises but also meditative practices that help in managing stress and enhancing the body's resilience.

TCM Perspective on EDC-Induced Health Issues
1. **Hormonal Imbalances**
   » TCM views hormonal imbalances as a disruption of yin and yang. Treatments focus on restoring this balance through a combination of acupuncture, herbs, and lifestyle modifications.
2. **Gut Health**
   » TCM recognizes the importance of a healthy digestive system for overall wellness. Practices like abdominal massage, herbal treatments, and dietary adjustments are used to enhance gut health.

Integrating TCM into Modern Lifestyles
1. **Consultation with Practitioners**
   » It is important to consult with qualified TCM practitioners who can provide personalized advice and treatments.
2. **Lifestyle Adaptations**
   » Incorporating aspects of TCM—such as mindfulness, moderate exercise, and a balanced diet—into daily life can be beneficial in mitigating the effects of EDCs.

Conclusion
The Chinese medicine perspective offers a valuable framework for understanding and combating the effects of EDCs. Its holistic approach, emphasizing balance, natural remedies, and the interconnection of body systems, provides a complementary path to conventional strategies in dealing with EDC exposure. Embracing these ancient practices in the context of our modern environment can lead to improved health outcomes and enhanced resilience against environmental toxins.

CHAPTER TWENTY-ONE:

Ayurveda's Holistic Approach to Mitigating EDC Impact

Ayurveda, the ancient Indian system of medicine, offers a holistic approach to health that encompasses physical, mental, and spiritual well-being. In the context of modern environmental challenges, including exposure to endocrine-disrupting chemicals (EDCs), Ayurveda provides insightful guidance on detoxification and balancing the body's innate energies. This chapter explores Ayurveda's perspective on mitigating the effects of EDCs through natural healing, diet, lifestyle changes, and herbal remedies.

Ayurvedic Principles in Combating EDCs

1. **Understanding Doshas**
   » Ayurveda is centered around the balance of three fundamental bodily energies, or doshas: vata, pitta, and kapha. Disruption caused by EDCs can be addressed by identifying and balancing these doshas through diet, lifestyle, and herbal treatments.

Understanding Doshas and Their Role in Detoxification

In Ayurveda, the concept of doshas—vata, pitta, and kapha—is central to understanding and treating health issues. These doshas represent different combinations of the five elements (earth, water, fire, air, and ether) and govern all biological, psychological, and physiological functions of the body, including detoxification. EDCs can disturb the balance of these doshas, leading to health issues.

- **Vata Dosha (Air and Ether)**
  » This dosha governs movement and is responsible for the elimination processes in the body. An imbalance can lead to issues like constipation or dehydration, hindering effective detoxification.
- **Pitta Dosha (Fire and Water)**
  » This dosha oversees metabolism and detoxification in the liver. Pitta imbalance can lead to inefficient processing of toxins and increased inflammatory responses.
- **Kapha Dosha (Earth and Water)**
  » This dosha regulates structure and fluid balance. An imbalance in the kapha dosha can cause sluggishness in the body's detox pathways, leading to accumulation of toxins.

2. **Detoxification (Panchakarma)**
  » *Panchakarma* is Ayurveda's primary purification and detoxification treatment, involving procedures like herbal oil massages, steam baths, and intestinal cleansing, designed to eliminate toxins from the body.

  Panchakarma, the intensive detoxification treatment in Ayurveda, is often customized based on the individual's dominant dosha and specific health needs, ensuring a balanced and effective detox process.

- **Vata Detoxification**
  - » This process focuses on nourishing and grounding treatments to stabilize the vata dosha. Practices might include warm oil massages (*snehana*) and gentle laxatives for cleansing.
- **Pitta Detoxification**
  - » This process is aimed at cooling and calming the pitta dosha. Therapies may involve consuming cooling herbs, purgation (*virechana*), and blood purification techniques.
- **Kapha Detoxification**
  - » This process involves stimulating and invigorating treatments to counter the kapha dosha's heaviness. Techniques include dry massages, steam therapy (*swedana*), and nasal administration of medicinal herbs (nasya).

3. **Strengthening Agni (Digestive Fire)**
   - » A strong *agni* is crucial for proper digestion and elimination of toxins. Ayurvedic practices recommend dietary and lifestyle changes to maintain a robust digestive system.

Ayurvedic Lifestyle and Dietary Adjustments for Dosha Balance

Ayurveda recommends specific lifestyle and dietary changes to maintain dosha balance, which is crucial for effective detoxification.

1. **Vata Balancing**
   - » Favor warm, cooked, nourishing foods. Engage in regular, grounding routines with gentle exercises like yoga, and avoid overstimulation.
2. **Pitta Balancing**
   - » Select cool, refreshing foods, and avoid spicy, hot dishes. Practice stress-relieving activities and ensure adequate rest.

3. **Kapha Balancing**
   » Choose light, warm foods, and incorporate invigorating physical activities into your daily routine. Avoid heavy, oily foods that can exacerbate kapha imbalance.
4. **Sattvic Diet**
   » Emphasize a sattvic diet, which is light, pure, and rich in prana (life force). This diet includes fresh fruits, vegetables, whole grains, legumes, and nuts, all of which can help counteract the effects of EDCs.
5. **Herbs and Spices**
   » Use specific herbs and spices, like turmeric, ginger, and cumin, which are known for their detoxifying and balancing properties.
6. **Avoiding Processed Foods**
   » Minimize the intake of processed and packaged foods that are likely to contain EDCs.

Lifestyle and Mind-Body Practices
1. **Yoga and Meditation**
   » Regular practice of yoga and meditation can help in managing stress, improving bodily functions, and enhancing overall resilience against environmental toxins.
2. **Daily Routines (Dinacharya)**
   » Adhering to a daily routine, as advised in Ayurveda, including waking up early, practicing oil pulling, and self-massage (*abhyanga*), can aid in maintaining balance and detoxification.

Ayurvedic Herbal Remedies
1. **Herbal Formulations**
   - » Utilize traditional Ayurvedic formulations like triphala, ashwagandha, and shatavari, which are believed to support detoxification processes and restore hormonal balance.
   - » **Herbal Support for Detoxification**
     - Depending on the dominant dosha and specific health needs, certain herbs are prescribed to support the detoxification process.
     - **Vata:** Herbs like ashwagandha and haritaki can be beneficial.
     - **Pitta:** Herbs such as amalaki and guduchi are often recommended.
     - **Kapha:** Pippali and trikatu are commonly used herbs.
2. **Customized Treatments**
   - » Ayurvedic treatments are highly individualized, based on one's dosha profile and specific health needs.
   - » Panchakarma, Ayurveda's primary purification and detoxification treatment, is tailored to individual dosha imbalances. It involves several phases.
   - » **Purvakarma (Preparation)**
     - This phase involves dietary changes and taking medicated ghee (clarified butter) to begin loosening the toxins.
   - » **Pradhanakarma (Main Procedures)**
     - This phase includes therapies like *vamana* (therapeutic vomiting) for kapha imbalance, *virechana* (purgation) for pitta, and *basti* (medicated enema) for vata.
     - Nasya (nasal administration of oils) and raktamokshana (bloodletting) may also be used.

» **Paschatkarma (Posttreatment)**
  - This phase involves restoring the digestive fire with a specific diet and lifestyle recommendations to maintain the detoxification benefits.

The Ayurvedic Approach to Modern Environmental Challenges

1. **Integrating Ayurveda into Everyday Life**
   » Explore practical ways to incorporate Ayurvedic principles into daily living for modern environmental health challenges.
2. **Environmental Consciousness**
   » Ayurveda also emphasizes living in harmony with nature, which aligns with reducing dependency on synthetic chemicals and EDC-laden products.

Conclusion

In Ayurveda, detoxification is not just a physical cleanse; it's a holistic process that involves balancing the doshas; nurturing the body, mind, and spirit; and realigning oneself with nature. Understanding one's predominant dosha and how it interacts with environmental factors like EDCs allows for a more personalized and effective approach to detoxification and overall health. By focusing on dietary and lifestyle modifications, stress management, detoxification processes, and the use of natural herbal remedies, Ayurveda offers a time-tested approach to restoring and maintaining health in the face of modern environmental challenges. Embracing these principles can lead to enhanced well-being, bringing balance and harmony to the body's natural rhythms amid the complexities of today's world.

CHAPTER TWENTY-TWO:

Naturopathic Remedies and Recommendations Against EDCs

Naturopathy, a holistic approach to wellness, emphasizes the healing power of nature and the body's inherent ability to heal and maintain itself. In the context of combating endocrine-disrupting chemicals (EDCs), naturopathic medicine offers a wealth of remedies and lifestyle recommendations. This chapter explores how naturopathic principles can be applied to reduce the impact of EDCs and promote overall health and well-being.

The Naturopathic Approach to EDCs
1. **First Do No Harm**
   » Avoidance of additional toxins is paramount. This principle involves choosing organic foods, using natural personal care products, and avoiding plastics.
2. **The Healing Power of Nature**
   » Emphasize foods and herbs that naturally detoxify the body and support hormonal balance.

3. **Identifying and Treating the Causes**
   » Address the root cause of any hormonal imbalances, which may involve reducing EDC exposure and supporting the body's detoxification processes.

Dietary Recommendations
1. **Organic Whole Foods**
   » Focus on a diet rich in organic fruits, vegetables, whole grains, and lean proteins to minimize exposure to pesticides and synthetic hormones.
2. **Cruciferous Vegetables**
   » Incorporate broccoli, cauliflower, brussels sprouts, and kale, which contain compounds that support liver detoxification.
3. **Fiber-Rich Foods**
   » Increase intake of fiber to aid in the elimination of toxins through the digestive tract.

Herbal Remedies
1. **Liver-Supporting Herbs**
   » Milk thistle, dandelion, turmeric, artichoke extract, and burdock root are known for their liver-supporting properties.
2. **Adaptogens**
   » Herbs like ashwagandha, rhodiola, and holy basil can help the body adapt to stress and support overall endocrine health.
3. **Detoxification Teas**
   » Green tea and herbal teas containing herbs like nettle, red clover, and cilantro can aid in detoxification.

Lifestyle Modifications
1. **Reducing Plastic Use**
   » Replace plastic containers with glass or stainless-steel alternatives, and avoid using plastic wrap and bottled water.
2. **Natural Personal Care Products**
   » Choose personal care products that are free of parabens, phthalates, and synthetic fragrances.
3. **Mind-Body Practices**
   » Incorporate stress-reducing practices like yoga, meditation, and deep breathing exercises.

Supplemental Support
1. **Antioxidants**
   » Supplements like vitamin C, vitamin E, and selenium can help protect the body from oxidative stress.
2. **Gut Health Support**
   » Use probiotics and prebiotics to maintain a healthy gut microbiome, which is essential for detoxification.

Environmental Awareness and Action
1. **Education**
   » Stay informed about the sources of EDCs, and actively participate in community and global efforts to reduce these toxins.
2. **Advocacy**
   » Support policies and initiatives that aim to reduce environmental toxins.

Conclusion

Naturopathy provides a comprehensive and holistic framework for dealing with the pervasive issue of EDCs. By combining dietary changes, herbal remedies, lifestyle adjustments, and environmental awareness, naturopathy offers practical and effective strategies for reducing the impact of these harmful chemicals. Embracing these principles can lead to improved health outcomes and contribute to a more sustainable and toxin-free lifestyle.

CHAPTER TWENTY-THREE:

Utilizing Essential Oils for Detoxification and Wellness

Essential oils, highly concentrated extracts from plants, have been used for centuries in various cultures for their medicinal and therapeutic properties. In the context of detoxification and countering the effects of endocrine-disrupting chemicals (EDCs), essential oils can offer significant benefits. This chapter explores how certain essential oils can be used to support the body's natural detoxification processes and promote overall wellness.

Essential Oils and Their Role in Detoxification

1. **Liver Support**
   » Certain oils (like rosemary, helichrysum, and carrot seed) are known for their liver-supporting properties. They can aid in enhancing the liver's natural detoxification capabilities.

2. **Supporting Kidney Function**
   » Juniper berry and geranium essential oils are believed to support kidney health, assisting in the natural elimination of toxins from the body.

3. **Lymphatic System Support**
   » Oils like grapefruit, lemon, and bay laurel are thought to support the lymphatic system, a key component in the body's detoxification process.

Application and Use of Essential Oils
1. **Topical Application**
   » Essential oils can be diluted with a carrier oil (like coconut or jojoba oil) and applied topically, especially over liver and kidney areas, or used in lymphatic massage.
2. **Aromatherapy**
   » Inhalation of essential oils using a diffuser or in a warm bath can promote relaxation, reduce stress, and support overall well-being, which is crucial during detoxification.
3. **DIY Blends for Detoxification**
   » Create custom blends tailored to individual needs for use in massages, baths, or diffusers.

Precautions and Safe Usage
1. **Quality Matters**
   » Always choose high-quality, pure essential oils from reputable sources to ensure safety and efficacy.
2. **Skin Sensitivity**
   » Perform a patch test before topical application to avoid allergic reactions, and always dilute essential oils with a carrier oil.
3. **Consultation with Professionals**
   » Seek advice from a certified aromatherapist or health-care professional, especially if pregnant, nursing, or dealing with specific health conditions.

Essential Oils for Stress Reduction
1. **Relaxing Oils**
   » Lavender, chamomile, and ylang-ylang can be particularly effective in reducing stress, a critical factor in holistic detoxification.
2. **Mood Balancing**
   » Oils like bergamot, clary sage, and frankincense are known for their mood-stabilizing properties.

Incorporating Essential Oils into Daily Routines
1. **Personalized Routines**
   » Incorporate essential oils into daily routines, such as using lavender oil in a bedtime routine for relaxation or lemon oil in morning rituals for an energizing start.
2. **Creating a Detoxifying Environment**
   » Regularly using a diffuser with detoxifying oils can help maintain a cleansing and rejuvenating atmosphere at home.

Conclusion
Essential oils can be a powerful tool in the journey of detoxification and wellness, offering a natural and holistic approach to combat the effects of EDCs. By understanding and harnessing their diverse properties, we can effectively integrate these potent plant essences into our daily routines, contributing to improved health and a more balanced lifestyle.

CHAPTER TWENTY-FOUR:

Vibrational Therapy to Promote Detoxification

Vibrational therapy, an alternative healing practice, revolves around the idea that the body has its own natural vibrational frequency which, when disturbed, can lead to imbalance and illness. This therapy uses sound, light, or electromagnetic fields to restore this balance and promote overall well-being. In the context of detoxification, especially with regard to countering the effects of endocrine-disrupting chemicals (EDCs), vibrational therapy offers unique methodologies to facilitate the body's natural detoxification processes.

Understanding Vibrational Therapy
1. **Principles of Vibrational Medicine**
   - » Vibrational medicine is based on the concept that all matter vibrates at specific frequencies, and that diseases and conditions are characterized by blockages or imbalances in these vibrations.

2. **Mechanisms**
   » It operates on the belief that the body can be brought back into a state of health by altering or tuning these frequencies.

Types of Vibrational Therapy for Detoxification
1. **Sound Therapy**
   » Sound therapy utilizes different aspects of sound, such as frequency, rhythm, and tone, to stimulate healing. Instruments like tuning forks, gongs, and singing bowls can be used to create therapeutic sounds.
2. **Color and Light Therapy**
   » These therapies involve exposure to specific colors or lights to balance energy in the body. Different colors are believed to correspond to different body systems and emotions.
3. **Electromagnetic Therapy**
   » This therapy uses electromagnetic fields to influence the body's energy flow. Techniques include pulsed electromagnetic field therapy (PEMF) and bioresonance therapy.

Implementing Vibrational Therapy
1. **Professional Guidance**
   » Seek out certified practitioners for personalized treatment plans, especially for more complex therapies like bioresonance.
2. **At-Home Practices**
   » Simple sound therapy practices, like listening to certain frequencies or using singing bowls, can be done at home to promote relaxation and detoxification.

3. **Integrating with Conventional Detox Methods**
   » Vibrational therapy can complement traditional detoxification methods, such as dietary changes and exercise, to enhance their effectiveness.

The Science Behind Vibrational Therapy
1. **Research and Efficacy**
   » While some aspects of vibrational medicine are supported by research, others remain more anecdotal in nature. It's important to approach these therapies with an open yet critical mind.
2. **Understanding Limitations**
   » Recognize that, while vibrational therapy can support detoxification and wellness, it should not replace conventional medical treatments for specific illnesses.

Safety and Precautions
1. **Consult Health-Care Providers**
   » Before starting any new therapy, especially if you have existing health conditions, consult with a health-care provider.
2. **Awareness of Overuse**
   » Avoid overuse or excessive exposure, particularly in therapies involving electromagnetic fields.

Conclusion
Vibrational therapy offers an intriguing and holistic approach to detoxification, aiming to harmonize the body's energies and promote healing. As we continue to explore innovative and integrative approaches to health, incorporating practices like vibrational therapy can be a valuable component of a comprehensive wellness plan, especially in combating the subtle yet pervasive impacts of EDCs.

CHAPTER TWENTY-FIVE:

To Detox or Not to Detox? Understanding the Pros and Cons of Detoxification Practices

A detoxification, often simply called a "detox," has become a buzzword in the world of health and wellness. It's commonly presented to purge the body of toxins, including endocrine-disrupting chemicals (EDCs). While some advocate for its benefits in promoting health and combating the effects of EDCs, others warn against potential risks and misconceptions. This chapter examines the advantages and disadvantages of various detox methods, offering insights into their efficacy and safety.

Understanding Detoxification

1. **Concept of detoxing:** At its core, detoxification is about assisting the body's natural processes in eliminating toxins. It can involve dietary changes, fasting, the use of supplements, and other methods.

2. **Removing accumulated targeted toxins:** Detoxification efforts are often aimed at removing specific toxins, including heavy metals, pollutants, and EDCs that accumulate in the body from the environment and lifestyle choices.
3. **Supporting the body's natural processes:** Detoxification practices are often aimed at supporting the body's natural detoxification systems, like the liver, kidneys, and lymphatic system.

Pros of Detoxification Practices

1. **Enhanced well-being:** Many individuals report feeling more energetic and mentally clear after a detox regimen.
2. **Lifestyle modifications:** Detox programs often encourage healthier eating and lifestyle habits, such as increased intake of fruits and vegetables, reduced consumption of processed foods, increased hydration, and regular physical activity.
3. **Improved digestive health:** Detox diets often lead to improved gut health due to the emphasis on high-fiber foods and probiotics.
4. **Enhanced organ function:** Some detox methods may support organ function, particularly of the liver and kidneys, which are critical for natural detoxification.
5. **Mental clarity and energy boost:** Many individuals report feeling more energetic, focused, and mentally clear during and after detox programs.

Cons and Criticisms of Detoxification Practices

1. **Lack of scientific backing:** Critics point out that many detox diets lack rigorous scientific evidence supporting their efficacy in toxin removal. The necessity and effectiveness of detox diets are often questioned by health professionals, as

the body naturally detoxifies itself through the liver, kidneys, and other systems.
2. **Potential nutrient deficiencies:** Some detox diets are extremely restrictive and can lead to nutrient deficiencies and muscle loss, causing more harm than good to the body.
3. **Potential health risks:** Some detox methods, especially those involving extreme fasting or use of laxatives, can be harmful, leading to electrolyte imbalances, dehydration, and digestive issues.

Safe and Effective Detoxification

1. **Consultations with health professionals:** Before starting any detox regimen, especially if there are underlying health conditions, consulting with health-care providers is crucial.
2. **Gentle detox methods:** Opting for milder detox approaches—such as incorporating more fruits and vegetables, avoiding processed foods, and staying hydrated—can be a safer way to support the body's detoxification.
3. **Lifestyle over quick fixes:** Incorporating detoxification as a regular aspect of a healthy lifestyle, rather than as a one-time or extreme event, can be more effective in the long run.
4. **Incorporating regular physical activity:** Regular exercise can enhance circulation and help the body's natural detoxification systems function more effectively.
5. **Eat foods that support detox of organs**
    » Dandelion root and greens
    » Lemon
    » Sauerkraut, kimchi, and other fermented foods
    » Sulphur-rich foods like eggs, broccoli, and kale
    » Apple cider vinegar
    » Chlorella and spirulina
    » Turmeric

6. **Intermittent fasting:** The 16/8 method involves fasting for sixteen hours then eating only during an eight-hour window. This activates the autophagy in the body, which clears your body of toxins down to the cellular level.
7. **Detox binders**
    » **Bentonite clay** has been used to remove lead and other toxins from the digestive tract.
    » **Chlorella/spirulina** detoxify the body from mercury and arsenic.
    » **Silica** can be used to detoxify from excess aluminum.
    » **Fulvic and humic acids** can remove pesticides and radioactive elements from the body.
    » **Activated charcoal** has been implemented to treat poisonings and drug overdoses.

The Role of Diet in Detoxification

1. **Whole foods:** A diet rich in whole foods, particularly those high in fiber, antioxidants, and essential nutrients, can support the body's natural detoxification processes.
2. **Hydration:** Adequate water intake is essential for detoxification, as it aids in digestion and nutrient absorption, and helps flush out toxins.

Detoxification Through the Lymphatic System: Removing Endocrine-Disrupting Chemicals (EDCs)

The lymphatic system is a crucial part of the body's detoxification process, working alongside the liver, kidneys, and other organs to remove toxins and maintain fluid balance. It is often referred to as the "drainage system" of the body, helping to eliminate cellular waste, pathogens, and harmful substances like endocrine-disrupting chemicals (EDCs). Understanding how the lymphatic system contributes to detoxification and how to support its function is essential for reducing the body's toxic burden and mitigating the harmful effects of EDCs.

Role of the Lymphatic System in Detoxification

The lymphatic system is a network of vessels, nodes, and organs that circulate lymph, a clear fluid that contains immune cells, nutrients, and waste products. This system plays a vital role in the removal of EDCs by the following processes.

1. **Transporting Toxins**
   » The lymphatic system collects toxins, including fat-soluble chemicals like EDCs, from tissues and transports them to the bloodstream, where they can be filtered and eliminated by the liver and kidneys.
2. **Immune System Support**
   » Lymph nodes filter lymph, trapping harmful substances like bacteria, viruses, and toxins. Immune cells in the nodes neutralize these threats, preventing them from circulating further in the body.
3. **Fat Transport and EDC Storage**
   » EDCs are often stored in fat tissues due to their lipophilic (fat-attracting) properties. The lymphatic system helps transport fats and fat-soluble toxins, aiding in their eventual elimination.

How Lymphatic Detoxification Assists in EDC Removal

1. **Reducing Toxic Load**
   » By clearing cellular waste and toxins from tissues, the lymphatic system prevents the accumulation of harmful substances like EDCs that could interfere with hormonal function.

2. **Enhancing Immune Function**
   » Efficient lymphatic drainage supports immune cell activity, which is essential for neutralizing the inflammatory effects of EDCs.
3. **Promoting Fat Metabolism**
   » Since EDCs are stored in fat, improving lymphatic function can support fat metabolism, indirectly reducing EDC storage and release.
4. **Supporting Tissue Health**
   » Proper lymphatic circulation prevents tissue stagnation, where toxins can accumulate and contribute to systemic inflammation and oxidative stress caused by EDCs.

Ways to Support Lymphatic Detoxification

Improving lymphatic circulation and function can significantly enhance the body's ability to eliminate EDCs. The following are some natural methods.

1. **Hydration**
   » Staying well hydrated ensures that lymph fluid remains thin and flows freely, allowing for efficient toxin transport.
   » **Action:** Drink eight to ten glasses of water daily. Add lemon to water for added detox benefits.
2. **Dry Brushing**
   » Dry brushing stimulates lymphatic flow by gently massaging the skin and encouraging lymph movement toward the heart.
   » **Action:** Use a natural bristle brush to gently stroke your skin in upward motions before showering.
3. **Exercise**
   » Physical activity, especially activities that involve muscle contractions, stimulates lymphatic circulation.

- » **Action:** Incorporate rebounding (jumping on a mini trampoline), yoga, or brisk walking into your daily routine.
4. **Lymphatic Massage**
   - » Manual lymphatic drainage (MLD) is a specialized massage technique that promotes lymph flow and reduces toxin buildup.
   - » **Action:** Seek a lymphatic massage professional, or perform self-massage techniques on key lymphatic areas (e.g., neck, underarms, groin).
5. **Dietary Support**
   - » Certain foods and nutrients can support lymphatic function and reduce the body's toxic burden.
     - Foods to include:
       - **Leafy greens (kale, spinach)** are rich in chlorophyll, which binds to toxins.
       - **Citrus fruits (lemon, orange)** contain antioxidants and vitamin C to support detox pathways.
       - **Garlic and ginger** are anti-inflammatory and promote circulation.
     - **Avoid** processed foods, refined sugars, and trans fats that impair lymphatic and liver function.
6. **Herbs and Supplements**
   - » **Cleavers (galium aparine)** supports lymphatic drainage and detoxification.
   - » **Echinacea** boosts immune function and helps clear lymphatic congestion.
   - » **Milk thistle** enhances liver detoxification, indirectly supporting lymphatic health.
   - » **Nettle tea** acts as a gentle diuretic to help flush toxins.

7. **Infrared Sauna Therapy**
   » Heat from an infrared sauna promotes sweating, which can aid in the release of toxins stored in fat and lymphatic tissues.
   » **Action:** Spend twenty to thirty minutes in an infrared sauna two or three times a week, ensuring proper hydration before and after.
8. **Deep Breathing Exercises**
   » The lymphatic system relies on body movements, including breathing, to circulate lymph. Deep diaphragmatic breathing stimulates lymphatic flow.
   » **Action:** Practice slow, deep breathing exercises (e.g., inhale for four seconds, hold for four seconds, exhale for four seconds) daily.

Alternative Approaches to Detoxification

1. **Mindful eating and regular exercise:** A balanced diet and regular physical activity can naturally support the body's detoxification processes.
2. **Stress management:** Techniques like yoga, meditation, and adequate sleep can help manage stress, which is crucial for optimal functioning of detoxification systems.

Conclusion

The decision to undertake a detoxification regimen should be an informed and balanced one, weighing the potential benefits against the possible risks. While detoxification can offer certain health benefits, it's important to approach these practices with a critical mind and ideally under professional guidance. Embracing a holistic and sustainable approach to health, which includes mindful nutrition, regular physical activity, and stress management, can naturally support the body's detoxification processes. This may be a more sustainable approach to maintaining long-term health and overall well-being.

CHAPTER TWENTY-SIX:

My Personal Journey

So I have shared a tremendous amount of information about EDCs, including how they cause disease and how to reduce their effects. I can imagine how overwhelming this may be. I, too, faced the daunting task of figuring out where and how to begin. I would like to share with you my own personal story and how I initiated my battle plan. Everyone is different, so I have previously outlined many options for you to choose from to create a personalized plan that works best for you. My first step was to have a comprehensive physical exam and evaluation by my primary care provider. I was found to have prediabetes with a HbA1c of 6.4 percent (normal is less than 5.6 percent). My cholesterol was normal at 189, but my bad cholesterol (LDL) was high at 132. My high-sensitivity C-reactive protein marker for inflammation was elevated at 2.1 mg/L (normal is less than 1.0). This put me at an average relative cardiovascular risk for heart attacks and strokes. My insulin was normal at 6 with a normal insulin resistance score of 12, which essentially ruled out insulin resistance. A few months later, I returned for reevaluation for upper stomach pains. A CT scan of my abdomen was performed, and my worst fears came to realization. I was diagnosed with a suspicious kidney tumor! Yes, it was quite a shock. Could I really have cancer? Nevertheless, with constant prayer and placing my faith and trust in God, I was able to face this new challenge. Thankfully, the tumor was small without spread, and it was treated successfully with cryoablation therapy which froze the tumor and caused it to die. My final biopsy was negative for cancer but noted "chronic inflammation." My belief, however, was that it had indeed been a cancerous or precancerous lesion that was healed by God. Nonetheless, the presence of chronic inflammation renewed my focus and energy to change my diet and lifestyle routine.

I then sought advice from a well-respected naturopath to dig deeper. I agreed to a full battery of nontraditional laboratory testing for heavy metals, toxins, and allergens. I would not recommend these to everyone, as they are quite expensive and are not covered by insurance. However, I personally found the results to be very informative as they pertained to my medical situation.

The first thing that was noted was an abnormal indican test. This was an indication of poor gut health as evidenced by poor protein digestion. As you can see, my score was severe for bowel toxicity.

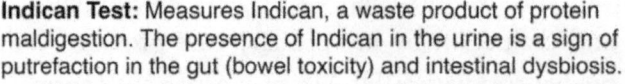

Indican Test: Measures Indican, a waste product of protein maldigestion. The presence of Indican in the urine is a sign of putrefaction in the gut (bowel toxicity) and intestinal dysbiosis.

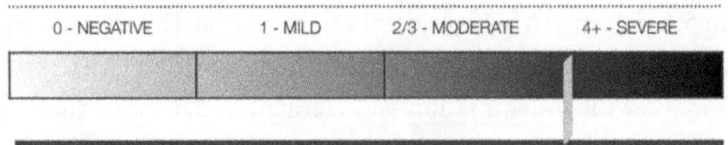

A food allergy test noted an intolerance to wheat or gluten, and to casein which is in many milk and dairy products. This explained the many stomach woes I have encountered when eating out at restaurants. I have switched to gluten-free options and to coconut milk and nondairy cheese substitutes.

```
Test Name                In Range    Out Of Range    Reference Range        Lab
WHEAT (F4) IGG                           6.0 H       <2.0 mcg/mL            SLI
    This test was performed using a kit that has not
    been cleared or approved by the FDA. The analytical
    performance characteristics of this test have been
    determined by Quest Diagnostics. This test, and any
    food specific allergen IgG result, should not be
    used for the diagnosis of allergic or atopic disease
    states (except for sensitivity to milk in neonates
    and gluten sensitivity). The use of food specific
    allergen IgG results should be restricted to the
    assessment of response to therapeutic interventions.
CASEIN (F78) IGG                        25.5 H       <2.0 mcg/mL            SLI
    This test was performed using a kit that has not
    been cleared or approved by the FDA. The analytical
    performance characteristics of this test have been
    determined by Quest Diagnostics. This test, and any
    food specific allergen IgG result, should not be
    used for the diagnosis of allergic or atopic disease
    states (except for sensitivity to milk in neonates
    and gluten sensitivity). The use of food specific
    allergen IgG results should be restricted to the
    assessment of response to therapeutic interventions.
```

My screen for heavy metals noted high levels of cadmium, nickel, zinc, thallium, silver, antimony, palladium, tin, and titanium. If you look at many of the labels of our personal care products, titanium dioxide is listed very often. I have now searched for makeup, sunscreen, and lotions that are free of this chemical. The palladium exposure was quite shocking to me. The major sources of exposure are from jewelry, dental crowns or bridges, the exhaust from cars, medical devise and other electronics, and food. To reduce exposure to palladium, wearing jewelry made from pure silver or gold, and getting routine dental exams, are recommended.

Toxic Element Exposure Profile; Hair

			TOXIC METALS	PERCENTILE
		RESULT µg/g	REFERENCE INTERVAL	68th 95th
Arsenic	(As)	0.036	< 0.14	
Lead	(Pb)	0.82	< 3.0	
Mercury	(Hg)	0.71	< 3.0	
Cadmium	(Cd)	0.089	< 0.20	
Chromium	(Cr)	0.64	< 0.85	
Beryllium	(Be)	< 0.01	< 0.050	
Cobalt	(Co)	0.036	< 0.15	
Nickel	(Ni)	1.2	< 1.0	
Zinc	(Zn)	370	< 300	
Copper	(Cu)	25	< 70	
Thorium	(Th)	0.002	< 0.005	
Thallium	(Tl)	0.004	< 0.005	
Barium	(Ba)	0.73	< 8.0	
Cesium	(Cs)	0.002	< 0.010	
Manganese	(Mn)	0.42	< 1.5	
Selenium	(Se)	0.79	< 2.1	
Bismuth	(Bi)	0.37	< 5.0	
Vanadium	(V)	0.028	< 0.20	
Silver	(Ag)	3.8	< 1.6	
Antimony	(Sb)	0.13	< 0.12	
Palladium	(Pd)	0.032	< 0.015	
Aluminum	(Al)	5.3	< 19	
Platinum	(Pt)	< 0.003	< 0.010	
Tungsten	(W)	0.004	< 0.015	
Tin	(Sn)	0.68	< 1.0	
Uranium	(U)	0.016	< 0.20	
Gold	(Au)	0.071	< 0.50	
Tellurium	(Te)	< 0.05	< 0.050	
Germanium	(Ge)	0.033	< 0.045	
Titanium	(Ti)	4.0	< 2.0	
Gadolinium	(Gd)	0.002	< 0.008	

Then I had an extensive screen for toxins and pesticides. Of note, I had moderate levels of triclosan which the FDA and EPA banned for use in hand sanitizers and hand soaps. However, for unclear reasons, it is still allowed in toothpastes, deodorants, makeups, cutting boards, and personal care products. Also noted were moderate levels of glyphosate from herbicides and pesticides, DMTP from contaminated foods, and phenyl glyoxylic acid from styrene and plastics. This is likely due to eating from restaurants with take-out containers that are often made from Styrofoam. Eating out also exposes us to many pesticides as it is cheaper to use nonorganic foods and products.

Environmental Toxins Summary

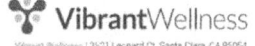

Moderate (75th-95th percentile)

TEST NAME	CURRENT RESULT	PREVIOUS RESULT	CURRENT RESULT	PREVIOUS RESULT	REFERENCE
Dimethylthiophosphate (DMTP)*	7.02		5.91	33.7	≤33.7 ug/g
Glyphosate	3.61		1.65	7.6	≤7.6 ug/g
Phenyl glyoxylic Acid (PGO)*	403.78		285	518	≤518 ug/g
Triclosan (TCS)*	43.47		29.9	358	≤358 ug/g

* Indicates NHANES population data reference ranges.

Urine Creatinine

TEST NAME	CURRENT RESULT	PREVIOUS RESULT	CURRENT RESULT	PREVIOUS RESULT	REFERENCE
Urine Creatinine	0.82		0.24	2.16	0.25-2.16 mg/mL

COMMENTS

Urine Creatinine

Urine tests that measure ratio of analytes by creatine concentration will not be altered by urine volume, hydration status, or time of testing. When using creatinine concentration to measure urine analytes, the only interference with the test is if the person's creatinine levels are very high (which may be seen in kidney disease, diabetes, or competitive body builder athletes), or when creatinine levels are very low (which may be seen in people with muscle wasting or sarcopenia who have lost their lean muscle mass stores). High urine creatinine may cause falsely lower urine analyte results. Low urine creatinine may cause falsely higher urine analyte results. This does not invalidate the findings; rather, critical analysis should be used to correlate results with clinical history and symptomatology for intervention decision-making.

TOXIC OVERLOAD: The Invisible Endocrine-Disrupting Chemicals Making Us Sick, Fat, and Tired

Environmental Toxins

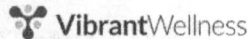

Vibrant Wellness | 3521 Leonard Ct, Santa Clara, CA 95054
1(866) 364-0963 | support@vibrant-america.com | www.vibrant-wellness.com

LAST NAME	FIRST NAME	GENDER	DATE OF BIRTH	ACCESSION ID	DATE OF SERVICE

Environmental phenols * Indicates NHANES population data reference ranges.

TEST NAME	PERCENTILE 75th 95th	REFERENCE	TEST NAME	PERCENTILE 75th 95th	REFERENCE
4-Nonylphenol	0.08	≤2.06 ug/g	Bisphenol A (BPA)*	1.52	≤5.09 ug/g
Triclosan (TCS)*	43.47	≤356 ug/g			

☐ COMMENTS

Triclosan (TCS)

Triclosan (TCS) is an antibacterial and antifungal agent present in some consumer products, including toothpaste, soaps, detergents, toys, and surgical cleaning treatments. Humans are exposed to triclosan through skin absorption when washing hands or in the shower, brushing teeth, using mouthwash, or doing dishes, and through ingestion when swallowed. Additional exposure is possible through ingesting plants grown in soil treated with sewage sludge or eating fish exposed to it. Triclosan has been associated with a higher risk of food allergies. Triclosan has also been found to be a weak endocrine disruptor. Prenatal triclosan exposure was associated with increased cord testosterone levels in the infants.

Herbicides * Indicates NHANES population data reference ranges.

TEST NAME	PERCENTILE 75th 95th	REFERENCE	TEST NAME	PERCENTILE 75th 95th	REFERENCE
2,4-Dichlorophenoxyacetic Acid (2,4-D)*	0.03	≤1.55 ug/g	Atrazine *	<0.01	≤0.05 ug/g
Atrazine mercapturate*	0.02	≤0.05 ug/g	Glyphosate	3.61	≤7.6 ug/g

☐ COMMENTS

Glyphosate

Glyphosate is the most used herbicide worldwide, and its residues can be found in food, drinking-water, crops, animal feed, groundwater, rain, and air. Residues have also been found in the urine of 60-80% of the general population in the United States. Potential health harms linked to glyphosate-based herbicides include microbiome disruption, increased risk of celiac disease, endocrine disruption, reproduction and fertility effects, cardiovascular disorder, central nervous system dysfunction, learning impairment, anxiety, depression, and renal disease. In 2015 the IARC, the specialized cancer agency of the WHO, classified glyphosate as a Group 2A carcinogen. Non-Hodgkin lymphoma has been significantly associated with occupational exposure to glyphosate in the literature. Multiple myeloma has also been associated with glyphosate exposure. Mechanisms shown in pre-clinical research for carcinogenicity and other health harms include increased production of reactive oxygen species (ROS), DNA adduct formation, mutagenic effects, and chromosomal damage.

Environmental Toxins

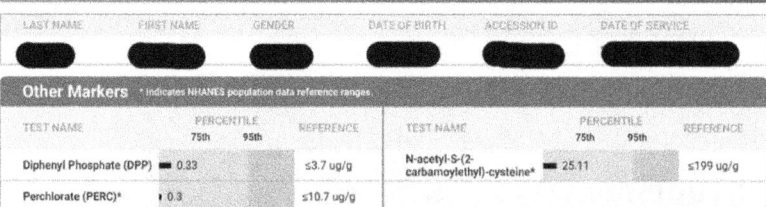

Other Markers *Indicates NHANES population data reference ranges.

TEST NAME	PERCENTILE 75th / 95th	REFERENCE	TEST NAME	PERCENTILE 75th / 95th	REFERENCE
Diphenyl Phosphate (DPP)	0.33	≤3.7 ug/g	N-acetyl-S-(2-carbamoylethyl)-cysteine*	25.11	≤199 ug/g
Perchlorate (PERC)*	0.3	≤10.7 ug/g			

Parabens *Indicates NHANES population data reference ranges.

TEST NAME	PERCENTILE 75th / 95th	REFERENCE	TEST NAME	PERCENTILE 75th / 95th	REFERENCE
Butylparaben*	0.07	≤4.39 ug/g	Ethylparaben *	0.03	≤99.3 ug/g
Methylparaben*	36.59	≤653 ug/g	Propylparaben*	8.41	≤222 ug/g

Pesticides *Indicates NHANES population data reference ranges.

TEST NAME	PERCENTILE 75th / 95th	REFERENCE	TEST NAME	PERCENTILE 75th / 95th	REFERENCE
2,2-bis(4-Chlorophenyl) acetic acid (DDA)	5	≤19 ug/g	3-Phenoxybenzoic Acid (3PBA)*	0.02	≤5.44 ug/g
Diethyl phosphate (DEP)*	0.9	≤15.7 ug/g	Diethyldithiophosphate (DEDTP)*	0.08	≤0.3 ug/g
Diethylthiophosphate (DETP)*	0.02	≤3.92 ug/g	Dimethyl phosphate (DMP)*	6.68	≤33.6 ug/g
Dimethyldithiophosphate (DMDTP)*	0.06	≤6.12 ug/g	Dimethylthiophosphate (DMTP)*	7.02	≤33.7 ug/g

COMMENTS

Dimethylthiophosphate (DMTP)

Dimethylthiophosphate (DMTP) is a metabolite of organophosphates, which are one of the most common causes of poisoning worldwide and are frequently intentionally used as pesticides. They can enter the body through the lungs or skin, or by eating contaminated food. Even at low levels, organophosphates may be hazardous to the nervous system, especially for foetuses and young children. Repeated or prolonged exposure may induce impaired memory and concentration, disorientation, severe depression, irritability, confusion, headache, speech difficulties, delayed reaction times, nightmares, sleepwalking, drowsiness, or insomnia. Organophosphates function by inhibiting the action of cholinesterase enzymes in nerve cells. An influenza-like condition with headache, nausea, weakness, loss of appetite, and malaise. Organophosphates and their metabolite, DMTP, generate oxidative stress, which in turn induces genomic instability through DNA damage. Alterations in genomic stability have been implicated in aging. Thus, DMTP may accelerate ageing owing to its contribution to genomic instability, which is a hallmark of aging.

Phthalates

TEST NAME	PERCENTILE 75th	PERCENTILE 95th	REFERENCE	TEST NAME	PERCENTILE 75th	PERCENTILE 95th	REFERENCE
Mono-(2-ethyl-5-hydroxyhexyl) phthalate (MEHHP)*	3.08		≤37.7 ug/g	Mono-(2-ethyl-5-oxohexyl) phthalate (MEOHP)*	2.64		≤23.4 ug/g
Mono-2-ethylhexyl phthalate (MEHP)*	2.39		≤8.47 ug/g	Mono-ethyl phthalate (MEtP)*	33.44		≤541 ug/g

Environmental Toxins

Vibrant Wellness | 3521 Leonard Ct, Santa Clara, CA 95054
1(866) 364-0963 | support@vibrant-america.com | www.vibrant-wellness.com

LAST NAME	FIRST NAME	GENDER	DATE OF BIRTH	ACCESSION ID	DATE OF SERVICE
▮▮▮	▮▮▮	▮▮▮	▮▮▮	▮▮▮	▮▮▮

Volatile organic compounds *Indicates NHANES population data reference ranges.

TEST NAME	PERCENTILE 75th	PERCENTILE 95th	REFERENCE	TEST NAME	PERCENTILE 75th	PERCENTILE 95th	REFERENCE
2-Hydroxyethyl Mercapturic Acid (HEMA)*	0.03		≤4.75 ug/g	2-Hydroxyisobutyric Acid (2HIB)	299.27		≤1215.72 ug/g
2-Methylhippuric Acid (2MHA)*	3.02		≤248 ug/g	3-Methylhippuric Acid (3MHA)	1.94		≤612.83 ug/g
4-Methylhippuric Acid (4MHA)	1.82		≤752.72 ug/g	N-Acetyl (2-Cyanoethyl) Cysteine (NACE)*	0.15		≤256 ug/g
N-Acetyl (2,Hydroxypropyl) Cysteine (NAHP)*	7.71		≤403 ug/g	N-Acetyl (3,4-Dihydroxybutyl) Cysteine*	0.2		≤583 ug/g
N-Acetyl (Propyl) Cysteine (NAPR)*	0.55		≤46.1 ug/g	N-acetyl phenyl cysteine (NAP)*	0.13		≤3.03 ug/g
Phenyl glyoxylic Acid (PGO)*		403.78	≤518 ug/g				

COMMENTS

Phenyl glyoxylic Acid (PGO)

Phenyl glyoxylic Acid (PGO) is a metabolite of styrene. Styrene is used in the manufacturing of plastics, in building materials, and is found in car exhaust fumes. Polystyrene and its copolymers are widely used as food-packaging materials. Styrene is a known carcinogen, especially in the case of eye contact. Long-term exposure to styrene may cause central nervous system and kidney effects, headaches, depression, fatigue, hearing loss, balance and concentration problems, and even cancer.

Lastly, I was screened for PFAS (per- and polyfluoroalkyl substances, also known as "forever chemicals"). What was so intriguing was that, even after removing all of my nonstick cookware, removing all plastic storage containers, and avoiding beverages in plastic containers, I still had moderate amounts detected in my urine. The likely culprit must have been from takeout foods, restaurant food containers, and water bottles. This proves that it is nearly impossible to avoid these toxins 100 percent of the time. However, we can maximize the body's capacity to detoxify and clear them from our system.

My Personal Journey

PFAS

Test Name	Current	Previous	Result (75th - 95th)	Reference
Perfluoroundecanoic acid (PFUnA) (ug/g)	1.098		0.695 - 1.267	≤1.267

POSSIBLE SOURCES

Contaminated food, Contaminated water, Polluted air, Firefighting foams, Detergents, Insecticides, Paper production, Food containers.

ASSOCIATED RISK

PFUnA and other perfluorinated chemicals can cause serious health effects, including cancer, endocrine disruption, accelerated puberty, liver and immune system damage, and thyroid changes. PFUnA exposure may lead to multiple glycerophosphocholines and fatty acids. PFUnA has the potential to generate reactive oxygen species (ROS), induce DNA damage and disturb the total antioxidant capacity (TAC) causing genomic instability. As genomic stability is the hallmark of ageing PFUnA can cause age associated conditions.

DETOX SUGGESTIONS

To detoxify PFUnA, individuals should strive to reduce exposure by avoiding contaminated water, food, and products containing perfluorinated compounds. Utilizing air purification systems can help minimize inhalation exposure. Supporting the body's natural detoxification mechanisms through adequate hydration, a nutritious diet, and regular physical activity may aid in eliminating PFUnA.

Creatinine

Test Name	Current	Previous	Result	Reference
Urine Creatinine (mg/mL)	0.73		0 - 0.24 - 2.16	0.25-2.16

PFAS

Test Name	Current	Previous	Result (75th - 95th)	Reference
Perfluorobutanoic acid (PFBA) (ug/g)	0.074		0.066 - 0.113	≤0.113

POSSIBLE SOURCES

Working in chemicals manufacturing and processing, Contaminated soil, Contaminated water, Personal care products, Cosmetics, Grease-resistant paper, Fast food containers or wrappers, Microwave popcorn bags.

ASSOCIATED RISK

Exposure to PFBA can cause peroxisome proliferation, peroxisomal fatty acid oxidation induction, and hepatomegaly. PFBA has the potential to generate oxidative stress and thereby induce DNA damage causing genomic instability. As genomic stability is the hallmark of ageing PFBA can cause age associated conditions.

DETOX SUGGESTIONS

To detoxify PFBA, individuals should prioritize reducing exposure by avoiding contaminated water, food, and products containing perfluorinated compounds. Implementing air filtration systems can help minimize inhalation exposure. Supporting the body's natural detoxification mechanisms through adequate hydration, a balanced diet, and regular exercise may assist in eliminating PFBA.

Test Name	Current	Previous	Result	Reference
Perfluorononanoic acid (PFNA) (ug/g)	0.871		0.652 - 1.31	≤1.31

POSSIBLE SOURCES

Possible routes of exposure to Perfluorononanoic acid (PFNA) include contaminated drinking water, contaminated food (especially fish), polluted air, exposure to fire-fighting foams, and contact with carpets and clothing. PFNA is detected in environmental media worldwide, with emissions from industrial facilities and precursor compounds like fluorotelomer alcohols (FTOH) contributing to its presence. Airborne transport of volatile precursors, such as FTOH, and long-distance transport via ocean surface currents are pathways for PFNA dispersion to remote areas.

ASSOCIATED RISK

High dose exposure to PFNA has long-lasting effects on the immune system. PFNA were found to induce sperm cell apoptosis. Increased serum lipids, primarily total cholesterol, LDL cholesterol, liver damage, neurodevelopmental effects, decreased weight of offspring are few symptoms of increased exposure to PFNA.

DETOX SUGGESTIONS

Regular administration of cholestyramine (CSM) resulted in the gastrointestinal elimination of different PFAS, including PFNA leading to a subsequent decrease in serum levels of all PFAS. However, additional investigation is necessary to grasp thoroughly the efficacy and safety of utilizing CSM therapy for detoxifying PFAS.

PFAS

Test Name	Current	Previous	75th — Result — 95th	Reference
Perfluorooctanoic acid (PFOA) (ug/g)	0.914		0.568 — 2.205	≤2.205

POSSIBLE SOURCES

Sources of exposure to perfluorooctanoic acid (PFOA) include contaminated drinking water, non-stick cookware, kitchen utensils, sealants, tapes, waterproof textiles, dental floss, leather goods, upholstered furniture, carpets, and rugs. Groundwater contamination can occur near sewage treatment plants, industrial sites, landfills, and locations where PFOA is used in firefighting foam. Additionally, fish and shellfish can accumulate PFOA from contaminated water, potentially impacting the food chain.

ASSOCIATED RISK

PFOA is a suspected endocrine disruptor and a common environmental pollutant. PFOA exposure may lead to a variety of adverse effects, including hepatotoxicity, immunotoxicity, and developmental toxicity. PFOA can stimulate cell migration and invasion, showing its potential to induce neoplastic transformation of human breast epithelial cells. Symptoms of PFOA are likely to be conditions like thyroid disease, high cholesterol, ulcerative colitis, pregnancy-induced hypertension, changes in liver function and reduced immune response. Severity of PFOA exposure can lead to cancers especially kidney, testicular, and thyroid cancer.

DETOX SUGGESTIONS

Regular administration of cholestyramine (CSM) resulted in the gastrointestinal elimination of different PFAS, including PFOA leading to a subsequent decrease in serum levels of all PFAS. However, additional investigation is necessary to grasp thoroughly the efficacy and safety of utilizing CSM therapy for detoxifying PFAS.

Test Name	Current	Previous	75th — Result — 95th	Reference
Perfluorotridecanoic acid (PFTrDA) (ug/g)	1.557		1.263 — 3.96	≤3.96

POSSIBLE SOURCES

Contaminated food, Contaminated water, Dust, Non-stick cookware, Water-repellent fabrics, Stain-resistant carpets, and Firefighting foam.

ASSOCIATED RISK

Perfluorinated substances like PFTrDA can pose significant health risks, encompassing a range of adverse effects such as cancer, disruptions in the endocrine system, early onset of puberty, liver and immune system impairments, as well as alterations in thyroid function. These chemicals exhibit remarkable persistence in the environment and have the propensity to accumulate within the human body. Among young males, exposure to PFTrDA may lead to decreased estradiol levels and impairment of Leydig cell function. Pregnant women exposed to PFTrDA may face an increased risk of elevated 1-hour plasma glucose levels. Additionally, prenatal exposure to PFTrDA has the potential to disrupt lipid metabolism in newborns. Furthermore, PFTrDA has been shown to induce DNA damage, with implications for genomic stability. This association with genomic instability suggests that PFTrDA's toxicity could contribute to an acceleration in the aging process.

DETOX SUGGESTIONS

Detoxification of PFTrDA involves minimizing exposure by avoiding contaminated water, food, and products containing perfluorinated compounds. Employing air purification methods can mitigate inhalation exposure. Supporting natural detox processes through hydration, a balanced diet, and exercise may aid in eliminating PFTrDA.

PFAS

Test Name	Current	Previous	Result (75th – 95th)	Reference
GenX/HPFO-DA (ug/g)	0.998		1.045 – 6.689	≤6.689
9-chlorohexadecafluoro-3-oxanonane-1-sulfonate (ug/g)	0.118		0.472 – 2.75	≤2.75
Dodecafluoro-3H-4,8-dioxanoate (NaDONA) (ug/g)	0.017		0.372 – 1.916	≤1.916
Perfluoro-[1,2-13C2] octanoic acid (M2PFOA) (ug/g)	<0.005		0.45 – 2.054	≤2.054
Perfluoro-1-[1,2,3,4-13C4] octanesulfonic acid (ug/g)	0.013		0.645 – 2.68	≤2.68
Perfluoro-1-heptane sulfonic acid (PFHpS) (ug/g)	0.126		0.628 – 3.783	≤3.783
Perfluoro-n-[1,2-13C2] decanoic acid (MPFDA) (ug/g)	0.602		0.94 – 2.907	≤2.907
Perfluoro-n-[1,2-13C2] hexanoic acid (ug/g)	<0.005		0.091 – 0.325	≤0.325
Perfluorobutanoic acid (PFBA) (ug/g)	0.074		0.066 – 0.113	≤0.113
Perfluorodecanoic acid (PFDeA) (ug/g)	0.218		0.696 – 2.399	≤2.399
Perfluorododecanoic acid (PFDoA) (ug/g)	<0.005		0.54 – 1.769	≤1.769
Perfluoroheptanoic acid (PFHpA) (ug/g)	0.012		0.106 – 0.142	≤0.142
Perfluorohexane Sulfonic Acid (PFHxS) (ug/g)	0.039		0.113 – 1.681	≤1.681
Perfluorohexanoic acid (PFHxA) (ug/g)	<0.005		0.01 – 0.156	≤0.156
Perfluorononanoic acid (PFNA) (ug/g)	0.871		0.652 – 1.31	≤1.31
Perfluorooctane sulfonic acid (PFOS) (ug/g)	<0.005		0.658 – 3.215	≤3.215
Perfluorooctanoic acid (PFOA) (ug/g)	0.914		0.568 – 2.205	≤2.205
Perfluoropentanoic acid (PFPeA) (ug/g)	<0.005		0.193 – 0.731	≤0.731
Perfluorotetradecanoic acid (PFTeDA) (ug/g)	1.140		1.478 – 4.912	≤4.912
Perfluorotridecanoic acid (PFTrDA) (ug/g)	1.557		1.263 – 3.96	≤3.96
Perfluoroundecanoic acid (PFUnA) (ug/g)	1.098		0.695 – 1.267	≤1.267

My battle plan consisted of the following:
- I changed all plastic food containers to glass storage containers.
- I changed all plastic water bottles to steel water bottles filled with water filtered at home.
- I changed all makeup to clean products without phthalates or parabens.
- I changed shampoos, soaps, lotions, deodorants, and hand sanitizers to natural ones.

- I slowly, over time, changed all my nonstick pots and pans to stainless steel, cast iron, and enameled cast iron pans.
- I avoided touching receipts and opted for electronic ones to be sent to my email.
- I eventually changed my plastic Vitamix blender container to a stainless steel one.
- I bought as many organic fruits and vegetables as possible, with a focus on a Mediterranean diet where I increased my intake of carrots, cruciferous vegetables, and green, leafy salads.
- I eliminated all dairy except for feta cheese and goat cheese, and I substituted with plant-based cheeses and coconut milk.
- I limited my meat intake and opted for plant-based protein substitutes, and I increased my salmon intake.
- I replaced all cooking oils with coconut oil, avocado oil, ghee, and olive oil.
- I limited my intake of foods containing gluten, like crackers and breads, and changed to plant-based and gluten-free options. My carb options were mainly quinoa and sweet potatoes. Although, I must admit to the occasional cheat day for pizza.
- I reduced my alcohol intake, especially with mixed cocktails. However, I do still have a glass of red wine once a week.
- Based on the advice of my naturopathy, I had to eliminate all coffee and say goodbye to my beloved Starbucks Pumpkin Spice latte and dragon fruit refreshers.
- I changed my sweeteners to calorie-free, plant-based sweeteners like allulose or monk fruit.
- I implemented an intermittent fasting regimen whereby my eating period was eight hours (from 11:00 a.m. to 7:00 p.m.) and I fasted for sixteen hours (from 7:00 p.m. through the next morning until 11:00 a.m.). I tried to avoid all snacks, except for almonds, walnuts, and pumpkin seeds with cranberries.

- I purchased a countertop reverse osmosis water filtration system for my drinking water. It is the only way to drink water that is free of microplastics, PFAS, volatile organic compounds, bacteria, viruses, and heavy metals.

My daily routine with a focus on anti-Inflammation comprised of the following:
- A shot glass of olive oil with lemon juice every day
- Omega-3 supplements
- Probiotics
- Vitamin D supplement
- Milk thistle, turmeric, and dandelion supplements for liver support
- Fresh lemon water made in a blender
- Fresh vegetable juice with organic carrots, celery, ginger, turmeric, and parsley
- Moringa and green tea every morning
- Either a smoothie of berries, coconut water, and flaxseeds, or a bowl of unsweetened Greek or coconut yogurt with fresh berries and nuts
- One cup of warmed organic chicken or vegetable bone broth before every dinner
- Getting at least ten minutes of sunlight daily
- Walking for ten minutes daily
- Prayer and meditation every morning

Here are a few of my sample meal plans:

Breakfast
- Moringa/green tea or hibiscus/green tea during my fast
- Lemon water throughout the day.

Lunch
- Avocado toast on gluten-free bread with sliced boiled egg and microgreens
- Leafy green salad with chickpeas, cucumbers, tomatoes, feta, cranberries, pumpkin seeds, and salmon or tuna
- Quinoa with broccoli
- Cauliflower rice with salmon or tuna
- Organic coconut or Greek yogurt with fresh berries, nuts, and cranberries

Dinner
- Baked sweet potatoes with grilled chicken, onions, and bell peppers
- Beyond Meat sauce with mushrooms and onions over zucchini noodles
- Grilled chicken or grass-fed beef with turmeric rice, hummus, and vegetables
- Asian-style quinoa with egg, broccoli, and kimchi
- Beyond Meat sausage with onions, peppers, cauliflower, and quinoa
- Vegetable omelet with side salad and kimchi
- Roasted spaghetti squash with Beyond Meat sauce with mushrooms and onions
- Vegetable lasagna with gluten-free pasta and side salad
- Black bean soup with salad or turkey sandwich
- Grilled lamb or goat meat in sauce with green plantains and salad
- Spinach quiche with side salad
- Berry and coconut milk smoothie with flaxseed oil and protein powder

At Night
Before the start of my overnight fast, I would drink herbal tea with chamomile and dandelion tea, have a piece of dark chocolate, or eat a cup of chia pudding with berries.

As I first began this battle meal plan, I noticed increased cravings for pizza, hamburgers, wings, Starbucks coffee, and alcohol. It was as if my body was fighting against my efforts. I was pleasantly surprised that I did not have any cravings for sweets or desserts, but I did miss my ice cream. I won't lie to you; it was very difficult ignoring these temptations. What I came to realize was that those cravings for processed or junk foods were actually stemming from the bad bacteria in my gut. These evil pathogens cannot thrive in a healthy, low acidic, and anti-inflammatory environment, and so they send signals for us to feed our body's the opposite. I also noticed some mild withdrawal symptoms of headaches, joint aches, and a stuffy nose. However, with some willpower, determination, and prayer, I was able to push through. Over time, the cravings decreased, my fatigue improved, and my withdrawal symptoms resolved. You may be asking yourself whether I was 100 percent diligent to this program, I must be honest and admit to the occasional cheat days and the times spent celebrating birthdays with friends and family. The key is to incorporate more of the anti-inflammatory measures, heal the gut, repair the liver, and live a full and healthy life. We will never be perfect. I can't tell you how many times I've cheated when family has come to visit, or during holidays and celebrations. Rather, let us strive toward being our better selves. With a healthy and well-functioning gut and liver, our bodies are well equipped to remove toxins. For example, by implementing many of these healthy options, I have been able to successfully reduce my HbA1c, normalize my C-reactive peptide (the marker for inflammation), and even lose some weight. I must stress the importance of devising a plan tailored specifically for you and checking with your primary care provider before you execute your own plan. In the next chapter, I want to appeal to everyone to spread the word and demand that companies reduce toxin exposures in our food, water, air, and everyday products.

CHAPTER TWENTY-SEVEN:

Final Thoughts: Encouraging Ongoing Awareness and Action

The pervasive nature of endocrine-disrupting chemicals (EDCs) in our environment, consumer products, and food supply presents a significant public health challenge. Addressing this issue requires more than individual action; it necessitates a collective push for systemic change. This chapter explores strategies for raising awareness, catalyzing action, and advocating for policy reforms aimed at stricter regulations on EDCs and the promotion of safer, healthier environments.

1. **Understanding the Scope of the Issue**

Before effective advocacy can begin, a deep understanding of the problem at hand is essential. EDCs are not confined to a single industry or product type; they are found in everything from agriculture to consumer electronics. Their ability to mimic or interfere with hormonal signals can lead to a host of health issues, making the fight against EDCs a multifaceted endeavor.

2. **Raising Awareness**

Education and awareness are the bedrock of any advocacy movement. Efforts to inform the public about EDCs should aim to do the following:

- » **Demystify the science:** Simplify complex scientific concepts for a general audience, highlighting the mechanisms by which EDCs affect our health and the environment.
- » **Share personal stories:** Personal narratives can be powerful tools in illustrating the real-world impacts of EDC exposure and fostering empathy and urgency.
- » **Utilize multiple platforms:** Engage communities through social media, workshops, public speaking events, and educational materials distributed in schools and community centers.

3. **Mobilizing Community Action**

With a well-informed community, the next step is to mobilize collective action.

- » **Grassroots campaigns:** Organize local campaigns to address sources of EDC exposure in communities, such as advocating for pesticide-free zones or the removal of harmful chemicals from local schools.
- » **Citizen science projects:** Encourage community participation in monitoring environmental pollutants, providing tangible evidence to support advocacy efforts.
- » **Lifestyle changes as advocacy:** Promote practices that reduce EDC exposure, such as organic farming, using natural products, and reducing plastic use, as both personal health measures and political statements against the widespread use of EDCs.

4. **Advocating for Policy Change**

The ultimate goal of raising awareness and mobilizing action is to effect policy change.

- » **Policy research and proposals:** Collaborate with scientists, legal experts, and policymakers to draft proposals for stricter regulations on EDCs, grounded in the latest research.
- » **Public comment and testimony:** Participate in public comment periods and provide testimony at regulatory hearings, using the collective voice of the community to advocate for change.
- » **Building coalitions:** Form alliances with environmental, health, and consumer rights organizations to strengthen advocacy efforts, share resources, and coordinate campaigns.

5. **Navigating Challenges and Setbacks**

Advocacy is often met with resistance from powerful interests and can be subject to political and economic pressures. Persistence, flexibility, and strategic thinking are key to overcoming these obstacles. Advocates should be prepared to:

- » **Counter misinformation:** Develop strategies to effectively counter industry propaganda and misinformation campaigns.
- » **Adapt strategies:** Be willing to adapt advocacy strategies in response to changing political landscapes and emerging scientific evidence.
- » **Celebrate small victories:** Recognize and celebrate progress, no matter how small, to maintain momentum and morale.

The following are some recent victories in the news:

- » A groundbreaking research article published by Elsevier in May 2023 found that the expression of 73 percent of known cancer-associated genes seen in breast cancer shifted to normal profile after people lowered their exposure to phthalates and parabens. Switching to personal care products free of these toxins made an impact in as little as twenty-eight days. Quite impressive!
- » On June 17, 2024, the Endocrine Society joined delegations from several countries to develop proposals to establish a new science policy panel charged with helping to inform governments, companies, farmers, and environmental entities about managing chemicals, reducing waste, and preventing pollution.
- » In December 2024, the European Commission adopted a ban on BPA in all food-contact materials. This includes items such as canned foods, plastic drink bottles, and kitchenware. There is hope that the US may soon follow suit.

Conclusion

Encouraging awareness, action, and advocacy for stricter EDC regulations and safer environments is a formidable challenge, but it is also an opportunity to foster healthier communities and a more sustainable world. Through education, community engagement, and persistent advocacy, it is possible to drive the systemic changes necessary to reduce the impact of EDCs on public health and the environment. The journey toward a safer future requires the collective effort of informed citizens, dedicated activists, and responsive policymakers, united in their commitment to protect human health and the planet.

Glossary

Adaptogens: Natural substances that are believed to help the body adapt to stress and to exert a normalizing effect upon bodily processes.

Antioxidants: Compounds that inhibit oxidation, a chemical reaction that can produce free radicals, thereby leading to chain reactions that may damage the cells of organisms.

Bisphenol A (BPA): A chemical compound used in manufacturing polycarbonate plastics and epoxy resins, including food storage containers and water bottles, known for its endocrine-disrupting effects.

Bisphenol S (BPS): A chemical used as a replacement for BPA in many BPA-free products. However, emerging research suggests that BPS also exhibits endocrine-disrupting activity, as does BPA.

Cruciferous vegetables: Vegetables of the family Brassicaceae (also called Cruciferae), such as broccoli, cauliflower, cabbage, and brussels sprouts, known for containing beneficial nutrients that support detoxification processes.

Detoxification (detox): The physiological or medicinal removal of toxic substances from a living organism, including the human body, which is mainly carried out by the liver.

Di (2-ethylhexyl) phthalate (DEHP): A phthalate used as a plasticizer to make plastic more flexible, found in a variety of consumer products, including plastic packaging films, toys, medical devices, and vinyl flooring. It is known to cause reproductive toxicity and has been linked to hormonal disruptions.

Dichloro-diphenyl-trichloroethane (DDT): A synthetic pesticide that was widely used in agriculture before being banned in many countries due to its environmental persistence and potential to harm wildlife and humans.

Dioxins: A group of chemically related compounds that are persistent environmental pollutants (POPs). These are toxic chemicals that remain in the environment for long periods of time and can accumulate in living organisms. Dioxins are formed through combustion processes and are found throughout the world in the environment. They can accumulate in the food chain, mainly in the fatty tissue of animals, and are highly toxic, causing reproductive and developmental problems, damaging the immune system, interfering with hormones, and causing cancer.

Doshas: In Ayurvedic medicine, the three energies believed to circulate in the body and govern physiological activity. The three doshas are vata (wind/spirit/air), pitta (bile), and kapha (phlegm).

Electromagnetic therapy: A type of therapy that uses electromagnetic fields to treat certain conditions by stimulating the body's healing processes.

Endocrine-disrupting chemicals (EDCs): Chemicals that can interfere with endocrine (or hormone) systems at certain doses. These disruptions can cause cancerous tumors, birth defects, and other developmental disorders.

Essential oils: Concentrated hydrophobic liquids containing volatile chemical compounds from plants, used in aromatherapy and other alternative therapies for their supposed health benefits.

Gut dysbiosis: A condition with imbalances in the microbial communities residing in the intestine, which can affect the body's ability to effectively detoxify harmful substances.

Heavy metals: Metallic elements with high atomic weights or densities that can be toxic or poisonous at low concentrations. Examples include mercury, cadmium, arsenic, and lead.

Herbal medicine: The study or use of medicinal herbs to prevent and treat diseases and ailments, or to promote health and healing.

Liver function: The liver's role in detoxifying chemicals and metabolizing drugs, as well as making proteins important for blood clotting and other functions.

Lymphatic system: The network of organs, lymph nodes, lymph ducts, and lymph vessels that produce and transport lymph from tissues to the bloodstream, an important part of the body's immune system and detoxification process.

Naturopathy: A form of alternative medicine based on a belief in vitalism, which posits that a special energy called vital energy, or vital force, guides bodily processes such as metabolism, reproduction, growth, and adaptation.

Organic foods: Foods produced using methods that do not involve modern synthetic inputs such as synthetic pesticides and chemical fertilizers, do not contain genetically modified organisms, and are not processed using irradiation, industrial solvents, or chemical food additives.

Organophosphates (OPs): A group of synthetic pesticides that affect the nervous system by disrupting neurotransmitters. Commonly used in agricultural practices, they have been associated with neurodevelopmental delays and cognitive impairments.

Panchakarma: A set of five therapeutic treatments administered to the patient for the complete detoxification of the body, according to Ayurveda.

Parabens: A class of widely used preservatives in cosmetic and pharmaceutical products, known to mimic estrogen in the body's cells.

Per- and polyfluoroalkyl substances (PFAS): A large family of synthetic chemicals used in nonstick cookware, water-repellent clothing, stain-resistant fabrics, and some firefighting foams. Known for their persistence in the environment and in the human body, they are suspected to affect growth, development, reproduction, thyroid function, the immune system, and the liver.

Perfluorooctanoic acid (PFOA) and perfluorooctanesulfonic acid (PFOS): Part of the PFAS family, these substances have been used in the manufacture of nonstick cookware, stain-resistant carpets, and water-repellent fabrics. Both are persistent in the environment and have been linked to various health issues, including developmental delays in children, decreased fertility, increased cholesterol, and compromised immune function.

Persistent organic pollutants (POPS): They are also known as "forever chemicals." These toxic chemicals (such as DDT, PFOS, and PCBs) are resistant to degradation by natural processes. They can remain in the environment for extended periods of time. They can travel long distances and can accumulate in living organisms, causing various health problems including developmental issues and damage to the nervous system or immune system.

Phthalates: A group of chemicals used to make plastics more flexible and harder to break, often used in consumer products such as plastic packaging materials and cosmetics, known for their potential as endocrine disruptors.

Polybrominated diphenyl ethers (PBDEs): Flame retardants used in a variety of household items such as electronics, furnishings, and textiles to prevent fires. They have been found to disrupt endocrine activity and neurodevelopment.

Polychlorinated biphenyls (PCBs): A group of man-made organic chemicals consisting of carbon, hydrogen, and chlorine atoms. They were used in various industrial and commercial applications, including as coolants and lubricants in transformers, capacitors, and other electrical equipment, and are now banned in many countries due to their health risks.

Vibrational therapy: A form of therapy that uses mechanical vibration (sound, light, or electromagnetic fields) to attempt to treat diseases by rebalancing the body's energy or vibrations.

Common Myths and Misconceptions

1. **Myth:** If a product is on the market, it must be safe from EDCs.
   Fact: Regulatory agencies do their best to ensure product safety, but not all chemicals have been thoroughly tested for endocrine-disrupting effects before they are allowed on the market. Moreover, regulations vary significantly between countries.

2. **Myth:** Only high doses of EDCs are harmful.
   Fact: EDCs can be active at very low doses, and their effects can depend on the timing of exposure. For example, fetal exposure to EDCs can have significant impacts on development that may not be evident until later in life.

3. **Myth:** Natural products do not contain EDCs.
   Fact: While natural products are less likely to contain synthetic EDCs, they can still contain naturally occurring

compounds with endocrine-disrupting effects or may be contaminated with EDCs during processing.

4. **Myth:** EDC exposure is only a concern for women and children.
   Fact: EDCs can affect individuals of any gender and age. While certain populations (like pregnant women, fetuses, and children) are more vulnerable, EDCs can impact adult men's health, including increasing fertility issues and cancer risk.

5. **Myth:** Everything causes cancer.
   Fact: While it's true that many substances have been linked to an increased risk of cancer, not everything causes cancer. The carcinogenic potential of a substance depends on various factors including the dose, duration of exposure, and an individual's genetic predisposition. EDCs are of particular concern because they can interfere with hormone functions, which play a significant role in the development and progression of certain cancers. By understanding which substances have stronger links to cancer, and how exposure occurs, individuals can take practical steps to minimize their risks.

6. **Myth:** The problem's too complicated, and there's nothing I can do.
   Fact: Although the issue of EDC exposure can seem overwhelming due to its pervasiveness, individuals have the power to significantly reduce their personal exposure through informed choices. Simple actions—like opting for fresh, organic foods over processed ones, using glass or stainless steel instead of plastics, and choosing personal care and household

products free of known EDCs—can make a difference. Collective actions and consumer demand for safer products can also influence industry practices and regulations over time.

7. **Myth:** We are protected since all food and products are independently tested for safety.
   Fact: Not all products undergo rigorous independent testing for safety, especially for long-term effects like endocrine disruption. Regulatory bodies do set safety standards, but these can vary widely by country and may not always be up to date with the latest scientific findings. Additionally, the testing often focuses on single chemicals rather than the cumulative effect of multiple exposures. Consumers looking for assurance about product safety should look for certifications from reputable third-party organizations.

8. **Myth:** Non-GMO is the same as organic.
   Fact: While "non-GMO" (nongenetically modified organism) and "organic" are often used interchangeably in consumer conversations, they refer to different standards and certifications in food production. Understanding the distinction between the two is crucial for making informed choices about reducing exposure to harmful substances, including EDCs.
   Non-GMO: This label indicates that the product does not contain genetically modified organisms. The focus is specifically on the genetic engineering aspect of food production. Non-GMO products can still be produced with conventional farming methods, which may include the use of synthetic pesticides, herbicides, and fertilizers that can contain or act as EDCs.

Organic: Organic certification encompasses a broader set of criteria than just the absence of GMOs. Organic standards, which vary by country but generally follow similar principles, prohibit the use of synthetic pesticides, herbicides, and fertilizers, as well as genetically modified seeds. Organic farming practices also emphasize soil health, biodiversity, and ecological balance, reducing the likelihood of EDC exposure from these products.

Key Takeaways

Organic products are inherently non-GMO, but they also meet additional requirements related to pesticide use, farming practices, and environmental preservation.

Non-GMO products do not guarantee the absence of synthetic pesticides or fertilizers that could contain EDCs.

Choosing **organic products** can be a more comprehensive approach for those looking to minimize their exposure to EDCs and support sustainable farming practices.

Frequently Asked Questions

1. **What exactly are EDCs, and how do they affect human health?**

    EDCs are chemicals, or mixtures of chemicals, that can interfere with any aspect of hormone action. They can mimic hormones, block hormone receptors, or alter the production and breakdown of hormones, potentially leading to a variety of health issues, including reproductive problems, developmental delays, metabolic issues, and increased cancer risk.

2. **Where are EDCs found?**

    EDCs can be found in a wide range of products, including plastics, personal care products, pesticides, electronics, and even in food and water supplies. They are also present in industrial waste and can accumulate in the environment.

3. **How long has the prevalence of EDCs been an issue?**

    The issue of endocrine disruption has been recognized in scientific and public health discussions for several decades, with increasing concern and research focus over time. The concept of chemicals interfering with the endocrine system, leading to adverse health effects, gained significant attention in the latter half of the twentieth century.

Early Observations
Instances of endocrine disruption in wildlife were noted as early as the 1950s and 1960s, with reports of reproductive and developmental abnormalities in fish and birds attributed to chemical pollutants in the environment. These early observations raised concerns about the potential for similar effects in humans.

Dioxin Research in the 1970s
Research on the toxic effects of dioxins, particularly TCDD (2,3,7,8-tetrachlorodibenzo-para-dioxin), in the 1970s provided early evidence of chemicals that could disrupt endocrine signaling pathways. Dioxins were linked to a range of health issues, including cancer, immune system suppression, and developmental problems, through mechanisms involving hormonal disruption.

DES Tragedy
Another early and tragic illustration of endocrine disruption in humans involved diethylstilbestrol (DES), a synthetic estrogen prescribed between the late 1930s and early 1970s to prevent miscarriages. It was later found to cause a rare type of vaginal cancer in daughters of women who took DES during pregnancy, as well as other reproductive issues, marking one of the first clear instances of endocrine-disrupting effects from synthetic chemicals in humans.

Rising Awareness in the 1990s

The publication of *Our Stolen Future* by Theo Colborn, Dianne Dumanoski, and John Peterson Myers in 1996 played a pivotal role in raising public and scientific awareness about endocrine disruptors. The book highlighted how everyday chemicals, from pesticides to plastics, could interfere with hormonal systems and cause various health and environmental problems.

Regulatory Actions

In response to growing evidence and concern, regulatory bodies and scientific organizations worldwide have taken steps to address endocrine disruptors. The European Union, for example, has been particularly proactive, implementing regulations to identify and control substances with endocrine-disrupting properties.

Today, the issue of endocrine disruption is widely recognized as a significant concern for public health and the environment. Ongoing research continues to uncover how EDCs can affect health by altering the functions of the endocrine system, influencing processes such as growth, development, metabolism, and reproduction. Efforts to better understand these chemicals, mitigate exposures, and develop safer alternatives are central to addressing the challenges posed by endocrine disruptors.

4. **How can I reduce my exposure to EDCs?**
   Reducing EDC exposure involves making informed choices such as using glass or stainless steel instead of plastic containers, choosing organic produce when possible, avoiding products with known EDCs like BPA and phthalates, and using natural personal care products.

5. **Are "BPA-free" products safe?**
   BPA-free products often use alternative chemicals that may have similar endocrine-disrupting effects. For example, BPS (bisphenol S) is frequently used as a BPA substitute but is also suspected of having similar health risks. Thus, a "BPA-free" label does not necessarily mean the product is risk-free.

6. **Are EDCs banned in the US and in the EU?**
   In the United States: The regulation of endocrine-disrupting chemicals (EDCs) in the United States is complex and varies by substance and use. The US does not have a comprehensive law specifically targeting EDCs as a unique class of chemicals. Instead, EDCs are regulated under various federal statutes and regulations, including the Toxic Substances Control Act (TSCA), the Federal Insecticide, Fungicide, and Rodenticide Act (FIFRA), and the Food, Drug, and Cosmetic Act (FD&C Act), among others. These laws empower agencies like the Environmental Protection Agency (EPA) and the Food and Drug Administration (FDA) to assess, regulate, and in some cases, ban or restrict the use of certain chemicals found to be harmful, including some EDCs. However, the regulatory approach often requires substantial evidence of harm before action is taken, and not all known or suspected EDCs are currently regulated or banned.

   In the European Union (EU): The EU has been more proactive than the US in identifying and regulating EDCs, employing a precautionary principle that allows for earlier intervention. Specific regulations, such as REACH (Registration, Evaluation, Authorisation, and Restriction of Chemicals) and the Biocidal Products Regulation, directly address the issue of EDCs and aim to protect human health and the environment from their effects. The EU has identified and banned or restricted the use of several substances known to be endocrine disruptors, especially in consumer products like cosmetics and pesticides. The European Chemicals Agency (ECHA) maintains lists of substances of very high concern (SVHCs), which include EDCs, and works toward limiting their use.

Comparison: The key differences between the approaches of the US and the EU lie in the regulatory frameworks and the principles applied in decision-making processes. The EU's use of the precautionary principle allows for more aggressive regulation of chemicals with suspected risks, including EDCs, whereas the US typically requires more definitive evidence of harm before taking regulatory action.

While both the US and the EU have mechanisms in place to regulate and control the use of harmful chemicals, including EDCs, their approaches and the extent to which EDCs are regulated or banned vary significantly. Advocates for public health and environmental protection continue to push for stricter regulations and more comprehensive policies to address the concerns associated with EDCs in both regions.

7. **Are all chemicals in products being tested for safety?**
While new chemicals are subject to safety testing before market approval, the testing does not always comprehensively evaluate potential endocrine-disrupting effects. For existing chemicals, which constitute the majority of chemicals in use, testing and regulation are even more challenging. Many have

been in use for decades, introduced before the understanding of EDCs and their potential health impacts. Not all chemicals in products are currently tested as safe regarding their potential to act as endocrine disruptors. There is a growing effort, particularly in regions like the EU, to improve the identification and regulation of EDCs. However, significant gaps remain in the testing, identification, and regulation of these chemicals globally. Consumers looking to minimize their exposure to EDCs are often advised to follow precautionary principles, such as choosing products with fewer and more natural ingredients and staying informed about the most recent scientific findings and regulatory updates.

8. **Can the effects of EDCs seen in laboratory testing be reversed?**
The question of whether the effects of endocrine-disrupting chemicals (EDCs) observed in laboratory testing can be reversed is complex and depends on several factors, including the specific EDC, the level and duration of exposure, and the biological system or organism being studied.

Type of EDC Exposure, Whether It Is Acute or Chronic
The reversibility of EDC effects can vary significantly between acute (short-term) and chronic (long-term) exposures. Short-term exposure may lead to reversible changes, especially if the exposure ceases and the body is given time to recover. In contrast, long-term exposure can result in more permanent alterations, particularly if critical developmental windows are impacted.

Timing of Exposure Dependent on Developmental Windows

Exposure to EDCs during sensitive periods of development (such as fetal development, infancy, and puberty) can have irreversible effects. For example, exposure to certain EDCs in utero has been linked to lasting developmental and reproductive issues. The timing of exposure is critical in determining the reversibility of the effects.

Organ-Specific Effects

The potential for reversal also depends on the specific biological systems affected. Some organ systems may have a greater capacity for regeneration and recovery, while others may sustain permanent damage from EDC exposure.

Intervention and Treatment

In some cases, interventions may mitigate the effects of EDCs. For instance, dietary changes, lifestyle modifications, and certain medications or supplements might help counteract some of the adverse effects of EDCs. However, the effectiveness of these interventions can vary widely.

Research Findings

» **Animal studies:** Much of what is known about the reversibility of EDC effects comes from animal studies. Some research has shown that removing the source of EDC exposure can lead to partial or full recovery in certain systems or end points, while other studies have documented irreversible effects, especially with exposures during critical developmental periods.

» **Human studies:** Evidence from human studies is more limited, but there are instances where reducing exposure to specific EDCs has been associated with improvements in health outcomes. For example, policy changes that reduce exposure to harmful EDCs have been linked to positive public health outcomes over time.

The potential to reverse the effects of EDCs observed in laboratory testing is highly variable and depends on a complex interplay of factors. While some effects, particularly those resulting from short-term exposures, may be reversible, others, especially those from exposures during critical developmental periods, may have long-lasting or permanent impacts. Ongoing research is crucial to fully understand these dynamics and develop effective strategies for prevention and intervention.

References

Chapter One

Cryer, P. E. "Glucagon in the Pathogenesis of Hypoglycemia and Hyperglycemia in Diabetes." *Endocrinology* 153 (3): 1039–1048.

De Felice, M., and Di Lauro, R. "Thyroid Development and Its Disorders: Genetics and Molecular Mechanisms." *Endocrine Reviews* 25 (5): 722–746.

Herman, J. P., McKlveen, J. M., Ghosal, S., Kopp, B., Wulsin, A., Makinson, R., and Myers, B. "Regulation of the Hypothalamic-Pituitary-Adrenocortical Stress Response." *Comprehensive Physiology* 6 (2): 603–621.

Knobil, E. "The Neuroendocrine Control of the Menstrual Cycle." *Recent Progress in Hormone Research* 36: 53–88.

Mullur, R., Liu, Y. Y., and Brent, G. A. "Thyroid Hormone Regulation of Metabolism." *Physiological Reviews* 94 (2): 355–382.

Muoio, D. M., and Newgard, C. B. "Mechanisms of Disease: Molecular and Metabolic Mechanisms of Insulin Resistance and Beta-Cell Failure in Type 2 Diabetes." *Nature Reviews Molecular Cell Biology* 9 (3): 193–205.

Röder, P. V., Wu, B., Liu, Y., and Han, W. "Pancreatic Regulation of Glucose Homeostasis." *Experimental and Molecular Medicine* 48 (3): e219.

Saper, C. B., Scammell, T. E., and Lu, J. 2005. "Hypothalamic Regulation of Sleep and Circadian Rhythms." *Nature* 437 (7063): 1257–1263.

Yen, P. M. "Physiological and Molecular Basis of Thyroid Hormone Action." *Physiological Reviews* 81 (3): 1097–1142.

Chapter Two

Bergman, Å., et al. "State of the Science of Endocrine Disrupting Chemicals 2012." *World Health Organization*.

Diamanti-Kandarakis, E., et al. "Endocrine-Disrupting Chemicals: An Endocrine Society Scientific Statement." *Endocrine Reviews* 30 (4): 293–342.

Endocrine Society. "Endocrine-Disrupting Chemicals (EDCs)." (n.d.).

Gore, A. C., et al. "EDC-2: The Endocrine Society's Second Scientific Statement on Endocrine-Disrupting Chemicals." *Endocrine Reviews* 36 (6): E1–E150.

Meeker, J. D., Sathyanarayana, S., and Swan, S. H. "Phthalates and Other Additives in Plastics: Human Exposure and Associated Health

Outcomes." *Philosophical Transactions of the Royal Society B: Biological Sciences* 364 (1526): 2097–2113.

National Institute of Environmental Health Sciences (NIEHS). "Endocrine Disruptors."

Rochester, J. R. "Bisphenol A and Human Health: A Review of the Literature." *Reproductive Toxicology* 42: 132–155.

United Nations Environment Programme (UNEP). "The State of the Science of Endocrine Disrupting Chemicals 2012."

Vandenberg, L. N., et al. (2012). Hormones and endocrine-disrupting chemicals: low-dose effects and nonmonotonic dose responses. *Endocrine Reviews*, 33(3), 378–455.

Zoeller, R. T., et al. (2012). Endocrine-disrupting chemicals and public health protection: a statement of principles from The Endocrine Society. *Endocrinology*, 153(9), 4097–4110.

Chapter Three

Bergman, Å., Heindel, J. J., Jobling, S., Kidd, K. A., and Zoeller, R. T. (Eds.). "State of the Science of Endocrine Disrupting Chemicals 2012." *World Health Organization.*

Diamanti-Kandarakis, E., Bourguignon, J. P., Giudice, L. C., Hauser, R., Prins, G. S., Soto, A. M., and Gore, A. C. "Endocrine-Disrupting Chemicals: An Endocrine Society Scientific Statement." *Endocrine Reviews* 30 (4): 293–342.

Gore, A. C., Chappell, V. A., Fenton, S. E., Flaws, J. A., Nadal, A., Prins, G. S., and Zoeller, R. T. "EDC-2: The Endocrine Society's

Second Scientific Statement on Endocrine-Disrupting Chemicals." *Endocrine Reviews* 36 (6): E1–E150.

Heindel, J. J., Newbold, R., Schug, T. T., and Zoeller, R. T. "Endocrine Disruptors and Obesity." *Nature Reviews Endocrinology* 11 (11): 653–661.

Küblbeck, J., Vuorio, T., Niskanen, J., Fortino, V., Braeuning, A., Abass, K., and Levonen, A. L. "The EDCMET Project: Metabolic Effects of Endocrine Disruptors." *International Journal of Molecular Sciences* 21 (8): 3021.

Trasande, L., Vandenberg, L. N., Bourguignon, J. P., Myers, J. P., Slama, R., and Zoeller, R. T. "Peer-Reviewed Research on Low-Dose Effects of Endocrine Disruptors." *Endocrine Reviews* 37 (4): 377–416.

Trasande, L., Zoeller, R. T., Hass, U., Kortenkamp, A., Grandjean, P., Myers, J. P., and Heindel, J. J. "Estimating Burden and Disease Costs of Exposure to Endocrine-Disrupting Chemicals in the European Union." *Journal of Clinical Endocrinology and Metabolism* 100 (4): 1245–1255.

Vandenberg, L. N., Colborn, T., Hayes, T. B., Heindel, J. J., Jacobs, D. R., Lee, D. H., and Myers, J. P. "Hormones and Endocrine-Disrupting Chemicals: Low-Dose Effects and Nonmonotonic Dose Responses." *Endocrine Reviews* 33 (3): 378–455.

Zoeller, R. T., Brown, T. R., Doan, L. L., Gore, A. C., Skakkebaek, N. E., Soto, A. M., and Vom Saal, F. S. "Endocrine-Disrupting Chemicals and Public Health Protection: A Statement of Principles from The Endocrine Society." *Endocrinology* 153 (9): 4097–4110.

Chapter Four

Akinbami, L. J., Cheng, T. L., and Kornfield, S. G. 2016. "Bisphenol A and Phthalates: How Environmental Exposures May Impact Pediatric Chronic Disease." *Journal of Clinical Endocrinology & Metabolism* 101 (12): 4855–48.

Bal-Price, A., Coecke, S., Costa, L., Crofton, K. M., Fritsche, E., Goldberg, A., and Wilks, M. F. 2012. "Advancing the Science of Neurodevelopmental Toxicity (NDT): Testing for Better Safety Evaluation." *Altex* 29 (2): 202–215.

Boccardi, V., and Herbig, U. 2012. "Telomerase Gene Therapy: A Novel Approach to Combat Aging." *EMBO Molecular Medicine* 4 (8): 685–687.

Braun, J. M., Kalkbrenner, A. E., Calafat, A. M., Bernert, J. T., Ye, X., Silva, M. J., and Lanphear, B. P. 2011. "Variability and Predictors of Urinary Bisphenol A Concentrations during Pregnancy." *Environmental Health Perspectives* 119 (1): 131–137.

Childs, B. G., Durik, M., Baker, D. J., and Van Deursen, J. M. 2015. "Cellular Senescence in Aging and Age-Related Disease: From Mechanisms to Therapy." *Nature Medicine* 21 (12): 1424–1435.

Chouhan, S., Flora, S. J. S., and Flora, G. "A systematic Analysis on Possibility of Water Fluoridation Causing Hypothyroidism." *Environmental Science and Pollution Research* 24 (7): 5841–5853.

Cooper, G. S., Parks, C. G., and Treadwell, E. L. 2009. "Occupational and Environmental Exposures as Risk Factors for Autoimmune Diseases." *Journal of Autoimmunity* 33 (3–4): 124–130.

Diamanti-Kandarakis, E., Bourguignon, J. P., Giudice, L. C., Hauser, R., Prins, G. S., Soto, A. M., and Zoeller, R. T. 2009.

"Endocrine-Disrupting Chemicals: An Endocrine Society Scientific Statement." *Endocrine Reviews* 30 (4): 293–342.

Firestein, G. S. 2003. "Evolving Concepts of Rheumatoid Arthritis." *Nature* 423 (6937): 356–361.

Franco, S., Blasco, M. A., and Sastre, J. 2017. "Environmental Stress, Telomeres, and Stem Cells: A Hazardous Link." *Frontiers in Genetics* 8: 147.

Harley, K. G., Gunier, R. B., Kogut, K., Johnson, C., Bradman, A., Calafat, A. M., and Eskenazi, B. 2013. "Prenatal and Early Childhood Bisphenol A Concentrations and Behavior in School-Aged Children." *Environmental Research* 126: 43–50.

Hauser, R., Meeker, J. D., Duty, S., Silva, M. J., and Calafat, A. M. "Altered Semen Quality in Relation to Urinary Concentrations of Phthalate Monoester and Oxidative Metabolites." *Epidemiology* 17 (6): 682–691.

Ho, S. M., Tang, W. Y., de Frausto, J. B., and Prins, G. S. 2017. "Developmental Exposure to Estradiol and Bisphenol A Increases Susceptibility to Prostate Carcinogenesis and Epigenetically Regulates Phosphodiesterase Type 4 Variant 4." *Cancer Research* 66 (11): 5624–5632.

Hotamisligil, G. S. 2006. "Inflammation and Metabolic Disorders." *Nature* 444 (7121): 860–867.

Kassotis, C. D., Stapleton, H. M., Kleinstreuer, N. C., Masse, L., and Demeneix, B. A. 2015. "Characterizing the Biological Activity of Chemicals Using an Endocrine Disruptor Screening Platform." *Toxicological Sciences* 148 (1): 112–127.

Khalil, A., Fenech, M., and Michael, H. 2018. "The Impact of Lifestyle, Diet, and Environmental Exposure on Telomere Length." *Genes* 9 (2): 77.

Khalil, A. B., Fenech, M., and Vassallo, M. T. 2018. "The Impact of Endocrine-Disrupting Chemicals on Skin and Hair: A Comprehensive Review." *Environmental Toxicology and Pharmacology* 62: 102–113.

Khanna, S., and Flora, S. J. S. "Assessment of Heavy Metal and Trace Element Levels in Patients with Chronic Telogen Effluvium." *Biological Trace Element Research* 154 (1): 22–28.

Kim, S., Park, J., and Kim, H. J. 2015. "Endocrine-Disrupting Chemicals and Ovarian Cancer: A Review of Recent Studies." *International Journal of Environmental Research and Public Health* 12 (8): 10206–10223.

Kim, Y., Ha, E. H., Park, H., Ha, M., Kim, J. H., Hong, Y. C., and Chang, N. 2017. "Prenatal Exposure to Phthalates and Infant Development at Six Months: Prospective Mothers and Children's Environmental Health (MOCEH) Study." *Environmental Health Perspectives* 125 (1): 149–154.

Landrigan, P. J., Sonawane, B., Mattison, D. R., McCally, M., and Garg, A. 2005. "Chemical Contaminants in Breast Milk and Their Impacts on Children's Health: An Overview." *Environmental Health Perspectives* 113 (10): 1359–1365.

Lee, S., Lee, J. S., Lee, H., and Kim, S. 2019. "The Role of Senescent Cells in Cancer and Age-Related Diseases." *Korean Journal of Internal Medicine* 34 (4): 1087–1098.

Libby, P., Ridker, P. M., and Hansson, G. K. 2002. "Inflammation in Atherosclerosis: From Pathophysiology to Practice." *Journal of the American College of Cardiology* 50 (9): 907–919.

Lyall, K., Croen, L. A., Sjödin, A., Yoshida, C. K., Zerbo, O., Kharrazi, M., and Windham, G. C. 2017. "Polychlorinated Biphenyl and Organochlorine Pesticide Concentrations in Maternal Mid-Pregnancy Serum Samples: Association with Autism Spectrum Disorder and Intellectual Disability." *Environmental Health Perspectives* 125 (4): 474–480.

Manikkam, M., Guerrero-Bosagna, C., Tracey, R., Haque, M. M., and Skinner, M. K. 2012. "Transgenerational Actions of Environmental Compounds on Reproductive Disease and Epigenetic Biomarkers of Ancestral Exposures." *PLoS ONE* 7 (2): e31901.

Manikkam, M., Tracey, R., Guerrero-Bosagna, C., and Skinner, M. K. 2012. "Pesticide Methoxychlor Promotes Epigenetic Transgenerational Inheritance of Adult-Onset Disease through the Male Germline." *PLOS ONE* 7 (3): e31901.

Martínez-Iglesias, O., Sánchez-García, D., Gómez-González, E., and Santamaría, R. 2010. "Phthalate Exposure Impairs Stem Cell Differentiation." *Journal of Cellular Biochemistry* 109 (5): 992–999.

Martens, D. S., and Nawrot, T. S. 2013. "Air Pollution and Cardiovascular Aging: The Role of Telomere Length." *Current Environmental Health Reports* 1 (2): 132–142.

Meeker, J. D., Calafat, A. M., and Hauser, R. 2011. "Urinary Bisphenol A Concentrations in Relation to Serum Thyroid and Reproductive Hormone Levels in Men from an Infertility Clinic." *Environmental Science & Technology* 44 (4): 1458–1463.

Palanza, P., Gioiosa, L., vom Saal, F. S., and Parmigiani, S. 2008. "Effects of Developmental Exposure to Bisphenol A on Brain and Behavior in Mice." *Environmental Research* 108 (2): 150–157.

Patisaul, H. B., and Bateman, H. L. 2008. "Neonatal Exposure to Endocrine Active Compounds or an ERbeta Agonist Impairs Female Reproductive Tract Function in Rats." *Frontiers in Neuroendocrinology* 29 (2): 162–172.

Pollard, K. M., Conrad, K., and Hudson, L. G. 2019. "Environmental Risk Factors for Autoimmune Diseases." *Current Opinion in Toxicology* 17: 13–23.

Prins, G. S., Tang, W. Y., Belmonte, J., and Ho, S. M. 2007. "Perinatal Exposure to Oestradiol and Bisphenol A Alters the Prostate Epigenome and Increases Susceptibility to Carcinogenesis." *Basic & Clinical Pharmacology & Toxicology* 102 (2): 134–138.

Rogers, J. A., Metz, L., and Yong, V. W. 2013. "Review of the Role of the Immune System in the Pathogenesis of Depression: Implications for Novel Therapeutic Approaches." *CNS Drugs* 27 (1): 5–15.

Rutkowska, A., and Rachoń, D. "Bisphenol A (BPA) and Its Potential Role in the Pathogenesis of the Polycystic Ovary Syndrome (PCOS)." *Gynecological Endocrinology* 30 (4): 260–265.

Sabanayagam, C., Teppala, S., Shankar, A. 2013. "Relationship Between Urinary BPA Levels and Prediabetes Among Subjects Free of Diabetes." *Acta Diabetologica* 50 (4): 625–631.

Selmi, C., Leung, P. S., Sherr, D. H., and Diaz, M. 2012. "Mechanisms of Environmental Influences on Human Autoimmunity: A National Institute of Environmental Health Sciences Expert Panel Workshop." *Journal of Autoimmunity* 39 (4): 272–284.

Sharma, A., Khera, A., and Paul, R. 2016. "Endocrine-Disrupting Chemicals and Skin Disorders: An Integrative Review." *Journal of Endocrinology* 231 (2): 73–87.

Skinner, M. K. 2014. "Environmental Epigenetic Transgenerational Inheritance and Somatic Epigenetic Mitotic Stability." *Epigenetics* 9 (8): 1153–1155.

Soto, A. M., and Sonnenschein, C. 2010. "Environmental Causes of Cancer: Endocrine Disruptors as Carcinogens." *Nature Reviews Endocrinology* 6 (7): 363–370.

Tabas, I., and Glass, C. K. 2013. "Anti-Inflammatory Therapy in Chronic Disease: Challenges and Opportunities." *Science* 339 (6116): 166–172.

Tanner, C. M., Kamel, F., Ross, G. W., Hoppin, J. A., Goldman, S. M., Korell, M., and Langston, J. W. 2011. "Rotenone, Paraquat, and Parkinson's Disease." *Environmental Health Perspectives* 119 (6): 866–872.

Thornton, M. J., Taylor, A. H., Mullally, R., et al. 2010. "The Role of Estrogen and Androgen Receptors in Human Scalp Skin." *Experimental Dermatology* 19 (4): 425–433.

Vandenberg, L. N., Hauser, R., Marcus, M., Olea, N., and Welshons, W. V. 2007. "Human Exposure to Bisphenol A (BPA)." *Reproductive Toxicology* 24 (2): 139–177.

Van Deursen, J. M. (2014). "The Role of Senescent Cells in Ageing." *Nature* 509 (7501): 439–446.

Vélez, M. P., Arbuckle, T. E., and Fraser, W. D. 2016. "Maternal Exposure to Perfluorinated Chemicals and Reduced Fecundity: The MIREC Study." *Human Reproduction* 31 (4): 821–828.

Wang, D., and DuBois, R. N. 2010. "The Role of COX-2 in Intestinal Inflammation and Colorectal Cancer." *Oncogene* 29 (6): 781–788.

Watson, C. S., Jeng, Y. J., Kochukov, M. Y., and Nanjappa, M. K. 2019. "Endocrine Disruption via Altered Gene Regulation and Environmental Signaling." *Frontiers in Endocrinology* 10: 211.

Zama, A. M., and Uzumcu, M. 2010. "Epigenetic Effects of Endocrine-Disrupting Chemicals on Female Reproduction: An Ovarian Perspective." *Frontiers in Neuroendocrinology* 31 (4): 420–439.

Chapter Five

Alonso-Magdalena, P., Morimoto, S., Ripoll, C., Fuentes, E., and Nadal, A. 2011. "The Estrogenic Effect of Bisphenol A Disrupts Pancreatic Beta-Cell Function in Vivo and Induces Insulin Resistance." *Environmental Health Perspectives* 119 (4): 402–409.

Claus, S. P., Guillou, H., and Ellero-Simatos, S. 2016. "The Gut Microbiota: A Major Player in the Toxicity of Environmental Pollutants?" *Biofilms and Microbiomes* 2 (1): 16003.

García-Arevalo, M., Alonso-Magdalena, P., Rebelo Dos Santos, J., Quesada, I., Carneiro, E. M., and Nadal, A. 2014. "Exposure to Bisphenol-A During Pregnancy Partially Mimics the Effects of a High-Fat Diet Altering Glucose Homeostasis and Gene Expression in Adult Male Mice." *PLoS One* 9 (6): e100214.

Grün, F., and Blumberg, B. 2009. "Endocrine Disrupters as Obesogens." *Molecular and Cellular Endocrinology* 304 (1–2): 19–29.

Hotamisligil, G. S. 2006. "Inflammation and Metabolic Disorders." *Nature* 444 (7121): 860–867.

Janesick, A., and Blumberg, B. 2011. "Endocrine-Disrupting Chemicals and the Developmental Programming of Adipogenesis and Obesity." *Birth Defects Research Part C: Embryo Today: Reviews* 93 (1): 34–50.

Lee, D. H., Porta, M., Jacobs, D. R., Jr., and Vandenberg, L. N. 2010. "Chlorinated Persistent Organic Pollutants, Obesity, and Type 2 Diabetes." *Endocrine Reviews* 31 (2): 202–229.

Sargis, R. M., Johnson, D. N., Choudhury, R. A., and Brady, M. J. 2010. "Environmental Endocrine Disruptors Promote Adipogenesis in the 3T3-L1 Cell Line Through Glucocorticoid Receptor Activation." *Obesity* 18 (7): 1283–1288.

Svensson, K., Hernández-Ramírez, R. U., Burguete-García, A., Cebrián, M. E., Calafat, A. M., and López-Carrillo, L. 2011. "Phthalate Exposure Associated with Self-Reported Diabetes Among Mexican Women." *Environmental Research* 111 (6): 792–796.

Thayer, K. A., Heindel, J. J., Bucher, J. R., and Gallo, M. A. 2012. "Role of Environmental Chemicals in Diabetes and Obesity: A National Toxicology Program Workshop Review." *Environmental Health Perspectives* 120 (6): 779–789.

Tuomisto, K., Jousilahti, P., Havulinna, A. S., Borodulin, K., Männistö, S., and Salomaa, V. "Role of Inflammation Markers in the Prediction of Weight Gain and Development of Obesity in Adults: A Prospective Study. *Metabolism Open* 3: 100016.

Chapter Six

Boas, M., Feldt-Rasmussen, U., Skakkebaek, N. E., and Main, K. M. 2012. "Environmental Chemicals and Thyroid Function." *European Journal of Endocrinology* 166 (5): 613–625.

Butt, C. M., Stapleton, H. M., Miranda, M. L., and Konstantinov, A. 2011. "Polybrominated Diphenyl Ethers (PBDEs) in House Dust and Beta-Glucuronidase Activity in Human Thyroid Cell Cultures." *Environmental Health Perspectives* 119 (1): 29–35.

Heindel, J. J., Blumberg, B., Cave, M., Machtinger, R., Mantovani, A., Mendez, M. A., and Vom Saal, F. S. "Metabolism Disrupting Chemicals and Metabolic Disorders." *Reproductive Toxicology* 68: 3–33.

Heindel, J. J., Newbold, R., and Schug, T. T. 2017. "Endocrine Disruptors and Obesity." *Nature Reviews Endocrinology* 13 (9): 536–546.

Meeker, J. D., Calafat, A. M., and Hauser, R. 2011. "Urinary Bisphenol A Concentrations in Relation to Serum Thyroid and Reproductive Hormone Levels in Men from an Infertility Clinic." *Environmental Science & Technology* 44 (4): 1458–1463.

Janesick, A. S., and Blumberg, B. 2016. "Obesogens: An Emerging Threat to Public Health." *American Journal of Obstetrics and Gynecology* 214 (5): 559–565.

Jumpertz, R., Le, D. S. N. T., Turnbaugh, P. J., Trinidad, C., Bogardus, C., Gordon, J. I., and Krakoff, J. 2011. "Energy-Balance Studies Reveal Associations Between Gut Microbes, Caloric Load, and Nutrient Absorption in Humans." *The American Journal of Clinical Nutrition* 94 (1): 58–65.

Küblbeck, J., Vuorio, T., Niskanen, J., Fortino, V., Braeuning, A., Abass, K., Rautio, A., Hakkola, J., Honkakoski, P., and Levonen, A. L. "The EDCMET Project: Metabolic Effects of Endocrine Disruptors." *International Journal of Molecular Sciences* 21 (8): 3021.

Lee, Y., et al. 2012. "The Association Between Endocrine Disruptors and Thyroid Nodules: A Clinical Study." *Journal of Environmental Health* 74 (9): 16–21.

Miyake, Y., Tanaka, K., and Arakawa, M. 2006. Household Pesticide Use and the Risk of Childhood Thyroid Cancer: A Population-Based Case-Control Study." *Environmental Health Perspectives* 114 (12): 1868–1872.

Paul, K. B., Hedge, J. M., DeVito, M. J., and Crofton, K. M. 2010. "Short-Term Exposure to Triclosan Decreases Thyroxine in Vivo via Upregulation of Hepatic Catabolism in Young Long-Evans Rats." *Toxicological Sciences* 113 (2): 367–379.

Pearce, E. N., and Braverman, L. E. 2009. "Environmental Pollutants and the Thyroid." *Best Practice & Research Clinical Endocrinology & Metabolism* 23 (6): 801–813.

Reynolds, A. C., Dorrian, J., and Liu, P. Y. 2017. "A Review of the Impact of Sleep on Gut Microbiota." *Current Sleep Medicine Reports* 3 (2): 78–85.

Ruhlen, R. L., Howdeshell, K. L., Mao, J., Bronson, F. H., and Newbold, R. R. 2011. "Low-Dose Exposure to Bisphenol A Alters the Plasma Levels of Thyroid Hormones and Pituitary Gonadotropins in Peripubertal Male Rats." *Environmental Health Perspectives* 119 (9): 1440–1445.

Zheng, X., Qiu, Y., Clark, J. M., and Bataller, R. 2020. "Pathogenesis of Nonalcoholic Steatohepatitis and the Role of the Gut-Liver Axis." *Liver Research* 4 (3): 141–149.

Zoeller, R. T., Dowling, A. L. S., and Herzig, C. T. A. 2007. "Thyroid Hormone, Brain Development, and the Environment." *Environmental Health Perspectives* 115 (8): 1261–1268.

Chapter Seven

Aguilera, M., Gálvez-Ontiveros, Y., and Rivas, A. "Endobolome, a New Concept for Determining the Influence of Microbiota Disrupting Chemicals (MDC) in Relation to Specific Endocrine Pathogenesis." *Frontiers in Microbiology* 11: 578007.

Ahima, R. S., and Flier, J. S. "Leptin." *Annual Review of Physiology* 62: 413–437.

Ahmadian, M., Suh, J. M., Hah, N., Liddle, C., Atkins, A. R., Downes, M., and Evans, R. M. "PPARγ Signaling and Metabolism: The Good, the Bad and the Future." *Nature Medicine* 19 (5): 557–566.

Blumberg, B. "Obesogens, Stem Cells and the Maternal Programming of Obesity." *Journal of Developmental Origins of Health and Disease* 2 (1): 3–8.

Claus, S. P., Guillou, H., and Ellero-Simatos, S. 2016. "The Gut Microbiota: A Major Player in the Toxicity of Environmental Pollutants?" *Biofilms and Microbiomes* 2 (1): 16003.

Darbre, P. D., and Harvey, P. W. "Paraben Esters: Review of Recent Studies of Endocrine Toxicity, Absorption, Esterase and Human Exposure, and Discussion of Potential Human Health Risks." *Journal of Applied Toxicology* 28 (5): 561–578.

Diamanti-Kandarakis, E., Bourguignon, J.-P., Giudice, L. C., Hauser, R., Prins, G. S., Soto, A. M., and Zoeller, R. T. 2009. "Endocrine-Disrupting Chemicals: An Endocrine Society Scientific Statement." *Endocrine Reviews* 30 (4): 293–342.

Drucker, D. J. 2005. "Biologic Actions and Therapeutic Potential of the Proglucagon-Derived Peptides." *Nature Clinical Practice Endocrinology & Metabolism* 1 (1): 22–31.

Engel, S. M., Buckley, J. P., Yang, J., Wu, M., and Herbstman, J. 2018. "Prenatal Phthalates and Childhood Adiposity in the Mount Sinai Children's Environmental Health Study." *Environmental Research* 162: 276–283.

Friedman, J. M. "Leptin and the Endocrine Control of Energy Balance." *Nature Metabolism* 1 (8): 754–764.

Fruebis, J., Tsao, T. S., Javorschi, S., EbbetsReed, D., Erickson, M. R., Yen, F. T., Bihain, B. E., & Lodish, H. F. (2001). *Proceedings of the National Academy of Sciences of the USA*, 98(4), 2005–2010.

Gálvez-Ontiveros, Y., Páez, S., Monteagudo, C., and Rivas, A. "Endocrine Disruptors in Food: Impact on Gut Microbiota and Metabolic Diseases." *Nutrients* 12 (4): 1158.

Giustina, A., Barkan, A., Casanueva, F. F., Cavagnini, F., Frohman, L., Ho, K. K., and Melmed, S. 2008. "Criteria for the Definition of GH Deficiency in Adults." *European Journal of Endocrinology* 157 (6): 695–700.

Gore, A. C., Chappell, V. A., Fenton, S. E., Flaws, J. A., Nadal, A., Prins, G. S., and Zoeller, R. T. 2015. "EDC-2: The Endocrine Society's Second Scientific Statement on Endocrine-Disrupting Chemicals." *Endocrine Reviews* 36 (6): E1–E150.

Gray, L. E., Jr., Ostby, J., Furr, J., Price, M., Veeramachaneni, D. N., and Parks, L. "Perinatal Exposure to the Phthalates DEHP, BBP, and DINP, but Not DEP, DMP, or DOTP, Alters Sexual Differentiation of the Male Rat." *Toxicological Sciences* 58 (2): 350–365.

Gribble, F. M., and Reimann, F. 2016. "Enteroendocrine Cells: Chemosensors in the Intestinal Epithelium." *Annual Review of Physiology* 78: 277–299.

Grün, F., and Blumberg, B. "Endocrine Disrupters as Obesogens." *Molecular and Cellular Endocrinology* 304 (1–2): 19–29.

Hampl, R., and Stárka, L. "Endocrine Disruptors and Gut Microbiome Interactions." *Physiological Research* 69 (Suppl 2): S211–S223.

Heindel, J. J., and Vandenberg, L. N. 2015. "Developmental Origins of Health and Disease: A Paradigm for Understanding Disease Cause and Prevention." *Current Opinion in Pediatrics* 27 (2): 248–253.

Heindel, J. J., and Blumberg, B. "Environmental Obesogens: Mechanisms and Controversies." *Annual Review of Pharmacology and Toxicology* 59: 89–106.

Höhn, C., Hahn, M. A., Gruber, G., Pletzer, B., Cajochen, C., & Hoedlmoser, K. (2024). Exposure to smartphone light suppresses melatonin levels at night. *Brain Communications*, 6(3), fcaf173.

Holst, J. J. 2007. "The Physiology of Glucagon-Like Peptide 1." *Physiological Reviews* 87 (4): 1409–1439.

Janesick, A. S., and Blumberg, B. "Obesogens: An Emerging Threat to Public Health." *American Journal of Obstetrics and Gynecology* 214 (5): 559–565.

Kadowaki, T., Yamauchi, T., Kubota, N., Hara, K., Ueki, K., and Tobe, K. "Adiponectin and Adiponectin Receptors in Insulin Resistance, Diabetes, and the Metabolic Syndrome." *The Journal of Clinical Investigation* 116 (7): 1784–1792.

Lehrke, M., and Lazar, M. A. "The Many Faces of PPARγ." *Cell* 123 (6): 993–999.

Marmugi, A., Lasserre, F., Beuzelin, D., Ducheix, S., Huc, L., Polizzi, A., and Guillou, H. "Adverse Effects of Long-Term Exposure to

Bisphenol A During Adulthood Leading to Hyperglycaemia and Hypercholesterolemia in Mice." *Toxicology* 325: 133–143.

Melzer, D., Rice, N. E., Lewis, C., Henley, W. E., and Galloway, T. S. 2010. "Association of Urinary Bisphenol A Concentration with Heart Disease: Evidence from NHANES 2003/06." *PLoS ONE* 5 (1): e8673.

Miyawaki, K., Yamada, Y., Ban, N., Ihara, Y., Tsukiyama, K., Zhou, H., and Seino, Y. "Inhibition of Gastric Inhibitory Polypeptide Signaling Prevents Obesity." *Nature Medicine* 8 (7): 738–742.

Newbold, R. R., Padilla-Banks, E., and Jefferson, W. N. 2009. "Environmental Estrogens and Obesity." *Molecular and Cellular Endocrinology* 304 (1–2): 84–89.

Newbold, R. R., Padilla-Banks, E., Snyder, R. J., and Jefferson, W. N. "Developmental Exposure to Endocrine Disruptors and the Obesity Epidemic." *Reproductive Toxicology* 27 (3–4): 273–282.

Ouchi, N., Parker, J. L., Lugus, J. J., and Walsh, K. "Adiponectin as an Anti-Inflammatory Factor." *Clinica Chimica Acta* 412 (1–2): 1–7.

Patisaul, H. B., and Bateman, H. L. 2008. "Neonatal Exposure to Endocrine Active Compounds or an ERbeta Agonist Impairs Female Reproductive Tract Function in Rats." *Frontiers in Neuroendocrinology* 29 (2): 162–172.

Rochester, J. R. "Bisphenol A and Human Health: A Review of the Literature." *Reproductive Toxicology* 42: 132–155.

Rosenfeld, C. S. 2017. "Gut Dysbiosis in Animals Due to Environmental Chemical Exposures." *Frontiers in Cellular and Infection Microbiology* 7: 396.

Rubin, B. S. 2011. "Bisphenol A: An Endocrine Disruptor with Widespread Exposure and Multiple Effects." *Journal of Steroid Biochemistry and Molecular Biology* 127 (1–2): 27–34.

Ruhlen, R. L., Howdeshell, K. L., Mao, J., Bronson, F. H., and Newbold, R. R. 2011. "Low-Dose Exposure to Bisphenol A Alters the Plasma Levels of Thyroid Hormones and Pituitary Gonadotropins in Peripubertal Male Rats." *Environmental Health Perspectives* 119 (4): 402–409.

Safe, S. H. "Endocrine Disruptors and Human Health: Is There a Problem?" *Toxicology* 205 (1): 3–10.

Sargis, R. M. 2014. "Environmental Endocrine Disruption of Energy Metabolism and Cardiovascular Risk." *Current Diabetes Reports* 14 (6): 494.

Sargis, R. M., Johnson, D. N., Choudhury, R. A., and Brady, M. J. 2010. "Environmental Endocrine Disruptors Promote Adipogenesis in the 3T3-L1 Cell Line Through Glucocorticoid Receptor Activation." *Obesity* 18 (7): 1283–1288.

Schug, T. T., Janesick, A., Blumberg, B., and Heindel, J. J. 2011. "Endocrine Disrupting Chemicals and Disease Susceptibility." *The Journal of Steroid Biochemistry and Molecular Biology* 127 (3–5): 204–215.

Shannon, M., Green, B., Willars, G., Wilson, J., Matthews, N., Lamb, J., Gillespie, A., and Connolly, L. "The Endocrine Disrupting Potential of Monosodium Glutamate (MSG) on Secretion of the Glucagon-Like-Peptide-1 (GLP-1) Gut Hormone and GLP-1 Receptor Interaction." *Toxicology Letters* 265: 97–105.

Sharpe, R. M. "Environmental/Lifestyle Effects on Spermatogenesis." *Philosophical Transactions of the Royal Society B: Biological Sciences* 365 (1546): 1697–1712.

Thaler, J. P., Yi, C. X., Schur, E. A., et al. 2012. "Obesity Is Associated with Hypothalamic Injury in Rodents and Humans." *Journal of Clinical Investigation* 122 (1): 153–162.

Tontonoz, P., and Spiegelman, B. M. "Fat and Beyond: The Diverse Biology of PPARγ." *Annual Review of Biochemistry* 77: 289–312.

Vandenberg, L. N., Colborn, T., Hayes, T. B., Heindel, J. J., Jacobs, D. R., Jr., Lee, D. H., and Myers, J. P. "Hormones and Endocrine-Disrupting Chemicals: Low-Dose Effects and Nonmonotonic Dose Responses." *Endocrine Reviews* 33 (3): 378–455.

Velmurugan, G., Ramprasath, T., Gilles, M., Swaminathan, K., and Ramasamy, S. "Gut Microbiota, Endocrine-Disrupting Chemicals, and the Diabetes Epidemic." *Trends in Endocrinology and Metabolism* 28 (8): 612–625.

Vom Saal, F. S., and Myers, J. P. "Bisphenol A and Risk of Metabolic Disorders." *Journal of the American Medical Association* 300 (11): 1353–1355.

Wada, N., Miyashita, A., and Shimizu, T. 2007. "Effects of Bisphenol A Exposure on the Proliferation and Apoptosis of Pituitary Cells in Vitro." *Toxicology in Vitro* 21 (5): 855–860.

Zhang, Y., Proenca, R., Maffei, M., Barone, M., Leopold, L., and Friedman, J. M. "Positional Cloning of the Mouse Obese Gene and Its Human Homologue." *Nature* 372 (6505): 425–432.

Zoeller, R. T., Brown, T. R., Doan, L. L., Gore, A. C., Skakkebaek, N. E., Soto, A. M., and Vom Saal, F. S. "Endocrine-Disrupting Chemicals and Public Health Protection: A Statement of Principles from The Endocrine Society." *Endocrinology* 153 (9): 4097–4110.

Chapter Eight

Ajao, C., Andersson, H., Hallberg, M., and Piersma, A. H. 2015. "Triclosan Inhibits Complex II and III of the Mitochondrial Electron Transport Chain." *Toxicology and Applied Pharmacology* 287 (1): 123–131.

Boas, M., Feldt-Rasmussen, U., Skakkebaek, N. E., and Main, K. M. 2012. "Environmental Chemicals and Thyroid Function." *European Journal of Endocrinology* 166 (5): 613–625.

Fujimoto, N., Tokunaga, T., Takada, H., and Endo, S. 2013. "BPA Inhibits Mitochondrial Biogenesis in Human Adipocytes." *Toxicology Letters* 218 (1): 121–126.

Heindel, J. J., Newbold, R., and Schug, T. T. 2017. "Endocrine Disruptors and Obesity." *Nature Reviews Endocrinology* 13 (9): 536–546.

Janesick, A. S., and Blumberg, B. 2016. "Obesogens: An Emerging Threat to Public Health." *American Journal of Obstetrics and Gynecology* 214 (5): 559–565.

Jumpertz, R., Le, D. S. N. T., Turnbaugh, P. J., Trinidad, C., Bogardus, C., Gordon, J. I., and Krakoff, J. 2011. "Energy-Balance Studies Reveal Associations Between Gut Microbes, Caloric Load, and Nutrient Absorption in Humans." *The American Journal of Clinical Nutrition* 94 (1): 58–65.

Kloas, W., Urbatzka, R., Opitz, R., and Ziková, A. 2009. "Endocrine Disruptors and Oxidative Stress." *Molecular and Cellular Endocrinology* 304 (1–2): 29–38.

Meeker, J. D., Calafat, A. M., and Hauser, R. 2011. "Urinary Bisphenol A Concentrations in Relation to Serum Thyroid and Reproductive Hormone Levels in Men from an Infertility Clinic." *Environmental Science & Technology* 44 (4): 1458–1463.

Reynolds, A. C., Dorrian, J., and Liu, P. Y. 2017. "A Review of the Impact of Sleep on Gut Microbiota." *Current Sleep Medicine Reports* 3 (2): 78–85.

Rüegg, J., Nilsson, S., and Henkel, C. 2017. "Epigenetic Effects of Endocrine-Disrupting Chemicals." *Molecular and Cellular Endocrinology* 448: 8–15.

Ruhlen, R. L., Howdeshell, K. L., Mao, J., Bronson, F. H., and Newbold, R. R. 2011. "Low-Dose Exposure to Bisphenol A Alters the Plasma Levels of Thyroid Hormones and Pituitary Gonadotropins in Peripubertal Male Rats." *Environmental Health Perspectives* 119 (9): 1440–1445.

Shen, H., Main, K. M., Virtanen, H. E., Damggard, I. N., Haavisto, A. M., and Toppari, J. 2014. "Endocrine Disruptors and Mitochondrial DNA Damage." *Environmental Health Perspectives* 122 (4): 395–403.

Zheng, X., Qiu, Y., Clark, J. M., and Bataller, R. 2020. "Pathogenesis of Nonalcoholic Steatohepatitis and the Role of the Gut-Liver Axis." *Liver Research* 4 (3): 141–149.

Chapter Nine

Bellanger, M., Demeneix, B., Grandjean, P., Zoeller, R. T., and Trasande, L. 2015. "Neurobehavioral Deficits, Diseases, and Associated Costs of Exposure to Endocrine-Disrupting Chemicals in the European Union." The *Journal of Clinical Endocrinology and Metabolism*, 100 (4): 1256–1266.

Bergman, Å., Heindel, J. J., Jobling, S., Kidd, K. A., and Zoeller, R. T. 2013. "State of the Science of Endocrine-Disrupting Chemicals 2012." United Nations Environment Programme and the World Health Organization.

Gore, A. C., Chappell, V. A., Fenton, S. E., Flaws, J. A., Nadal, A., Prins, G. S., and Zoeller, R. T. 2015. "EDC-2: The Endocrine Society's Second Scientific Statement on Endocrine-Disrupting Chemicals." *Endocrine Reviews* 36 (6): E1–E150.

Harley, K. G., Berger, K. P., Kogut, K., Parra, K., Lustig, R. H., Greenspan, L. C., and Eskenazi, B. 2016. "Association of Prenatal and Childhood PBDE Exposure with Timing of Puberty in Boys and Girls." *Environment International* 94: 499–506.

Heindel, J. J., and Blumberg, B. 2019. "Environmentally Induced Metabolic Disorders." *International Journal of Obesity* 43: 1285–1294.

Toppari, J., Virtanen, H. E., Main, K. M., and Skakkebaek, N. E. 2010. "Cryptorchidism and Hypospadias as a Sign of Testicular Dysgenesis Syndrome (TDS): Environmental Connection." *Birth Defects Research Part A: Clinical and Molecular Teratology* 88 (10): 910–919.

Chapter Ten

Lee, W. M. 2012. "Acute Liver Failure." *Seminars in Respiratory and Critical Care Medicine* 33 (1): 36–45.

Sanyal, A. J., et al. 2019. "Pioglitazone, Vitamin E, or Placebo for Nonalcoholic Steatohepatitis." *New England Journal of Medicine* 362 (18): 1675–1685.

Stickel, F., and Schuppan, D. 2007. "Herbal Medicine in the Treatment of Liver Diseases." *Digestive and Liver Disease* 39 (4): 293–304.

Chapter Eleven

Camilleri, M. 2019. "Leaky Gut: Mechanisms, Measurement and Clinical Implications in Humans." *Gut* 68 (8): 1516–1526.

Cresci, G. A., and Bawden, E. 2015. "Gut Microbiome: What We Do and Don't Know." *Nutrition in Clinical Practice* 30 (6): 734–746.

Zhang, Y. J., Li, S., Gan, R. Y., Zhou, T., Xu, D. P., and Li, H. B. 2015. "Impacts of Gut Bacteria on Human Health and Diseases." *International Journal of Molecular Sciences* 16 (4): 7493–7519.

Chapter Thirteen

Cerf, M. E. 2013. "Beta Cell Dysfunction and Insulin Resistance." *Frontiers in Endocrinology* 4: 37.

Hartman, M. L., et al. 1992. "Augmented Growth Hormone (GH) Secretory Burst Frequency and Amplitude Mediate Enhanced GH Secretion During a Two-Day Fast in Normal Men." *The Journal of Clinical Endocrinology & Metabolism* 74 (4) 757–765.

Myers Jr., M. G., Cowley, M. A., and Münzberg, H. 2008. "Mechanisms of Leptin Action and Leptin Resistance." *Annual Review of Physiology* 70: 537–556.

Myers Jr., M. G., and Olson, D. P. 2012. "Central Nervous System Control of Metabolism." *Nature* 491 (7424): 357–363.

Rattan, S., and Zhou, C. 2014. "Endocrine Disruptors, Obesity, and Inflammation." *Endocrine, Metabolic & Immune Disorders Drug Targets* 14 (3): 152–163.

Stickel, F., and Schuppan, D. 2007. "Herbal Medicine in the Treatment of Liver Diseases." *Digestive and Liver Disease* 39 (4): 293–304.

Whirledge, S., and Cidlowski, J. A. 2010. "Glucocorticoids, Stress, and Fertility." *Minerva Endocrinologica* 35 (2): 109.

Zimmermann, M. B., and Boelaert, K. 2015. "Iodine Deficiency and Thyroid Disorders." *The Lancet Diabetes & Endocrinology* 3 (4): 286–295.

Chapter Fourteen

Rochester, J. R. 2013. "Bisphenol A and Human Health: A Review of the Literature." *Reproductive Toxicology* 42: 132–155.

Sathyanarayana, S. 2008. "Phthalates and Children's Health." *Current Problems in Pediatric and Adolescent Health Care* 38 (2): 34–49.

Swan, S. H. 2008. "Environmental Phthalate Exposure in Relation to Reproductive Outcomes and Other Health Endpoints in Humans." *Environmental Research* 108 (2): 177–184.

Talsness, C. E., Andrade, A. J., Kuriyama, S. N., Taylor, J. A., and vom Saal, F. S. 2009. "Components of Plastic: Experimental Studies on

Animals and Relevance for Human Health." *Philosophical Transactions of the Royal Society B: Biological Sciences* 364 (1526): 2079–2096.

Teuten, E. L., Saquing, J. M., Knappe, D. R., Barlaz, M. A., Jonsson, S., Björn, A., and Takada, H. 2009. "Transport and Release of Chemicals from Plastics to the Environment and to Wildlife." *Philosophical Transactions of the Royal Society B: Biological Sciences* 364 (1526): 2027–2045.

Vandenberg, L. N., Colborn, T., Hayes, T. B., Heindel, J. J., Jacobs Jr., D. R., Lee, D. H., and Welshons, W. V. 2012. "Hormones and Endocrine-Disrupting Chemicals: Low-Dose Effects and Nonmonotonic Dose Responses." *Endocrine Reviews* 33 (3): 378–455.

Yang, C. Z., Yaniger, S. I., Jordan, V. C., Klein, D. J., and Bittner, G. D. 2011. "Most Plastic Products Release Estrogenic Chemicals: A Potential Health Problem that Can Be Solved." *Environmental Health Perspectives* 119 (7): 989–996.

Chapter Eighteen

Burch, J. B., Reif, J. S., Yost, M. G., and Neri, F. 1999. "Melatonin Metabolite Excretion Among Cellular Telephone Users." *International Journal of Radiation Biology* 75 (4): 447–456.

Chevalier, G., Sinatra, S. T., Oschman, J. L., Delany, R. M., and Sense, K. S. 2012. "Earthing: Health Implications of Reconnecting the Human Body to the Earth's Surface Electrons." *Journal of Environmental and Public Health*.

Halgamuge, M. N. 2013. "Pineal Melatonin Level Disruption in Humans due to Electromagnetic Fields and ICNIRP Limits." *Radiation Protection Dosimetry* 154 (4): 405–416.

Hardeland, R. 2008. "Melatonin and the Electron Transport Chain." *Cellular and Molecular Life Sciences* 65 (4): 1163–1184.

Reiter, R. J., Tan, D. X., and Korkmaz, A. 2014. "The Circadian Melatonin Rhythm and Its Modulation: Possible Impact on Human Health." *Sleep Medicine Reviews* 17 (4): 343–352.

Chapter Twenty

Chen, J. K., and Chen, T. T. 2004. "Chinese Medical Herbology and Pharmacology." Art of Medicine Press.

Liu, Y., and Wang, H. 2007. "Recent Advances in the Understanding of Molecular Mechanisms of Toxic Effects of Endocrine-Disrupting Chemicals: Is Traditional Chinese Medicine Protective Against Endocrine Disruptors?" *Environmental Health and Preventive Medicine* 12 (5): 204–217.

Maciocia, G. 2015. *The Foundations of Chinese Medicine: A Comprehensive Text.* Elsevier Health Sciences.

Tang, Y., and Tsai, S. Y. 2018. "Evaluation of Traditional Chinese Herbal Medicine in the Treatment of Polycystic Ovary Syndrome." *Gynecological Endocrinology* 34 (8): 659–665.

Zhang, Q., and Yu, P. 2019. "The Role of Traditional Chinese Medicine in the Management of Chronic Kidney Disease." *Kidney Diseases* 5 (1): 18–28.

Chapter Twenty-One

Lad, V. 2002. *Ayurveda: The Science of Self-Healing: A Practical Guide.* Lotus Press.

Singh, R. H. 2017. "An Assessment of the Ayurvedic Concept of Cancer and a New Paradigm of Anticancer Treatment in Ayurveda." *Journal of Alternative and Complementary Medicine* 23 (10): 755–761.

Chapter Twenty-Two

Boon, H., and Smith, M. 2004. *The Complete Natural Medicine Guide to the 50 Most Common Medicinal Herbs.* Robert Rose.

Pizzorno, J. 2016. *The Toxin Solution: How Hidden Poisons in the Air, Water, Food, and Products We Use Are Destroying Our Health—and What We Can Do to Fix It.* HarperOne.

Chapter Twenty-Three

Buckle, J. 2015. *Clinical Aromatherapy: Essential Oils in Healthcare (Third Edition).* Elsevier Health Sciences.

Tisserand, R., and Young, R. 2014. *Essential Oil Safety: A Guide for Health Care Professionals (Second Edition).* Churchill Livingstone.

Chapter Twenty-Four

Ernst, E. 2009. *Homeopathy: The Undiluted Facts.* Springer.

Federal Trade Commission (FTC). (n.d.). Consumer Information on Health. Citation: The FTC provides guidelines and warnings about the marketing of health-related therapies, including vibrational therapies, emphasizing consumer safety and the importance of substantiating health claims.

Gerber, R. 2001. *Vibrational Medicine: The Number One Handbook of Subtle-Energy Therapies (Third Edition).* Bear & Company.

Goldsby, T. L., Goldsby, M. E., McWalters, M., and Mills, P. J. 2017. "Effects of Singing Bowl Sound Meditation on Mood, Tension, and Well-Being: An Observational Study." *Journal of Evidence-Based Complementary & Alternative Medicine* 22 (3): 401–406.

Markov, M. S. (2007). "Expanding Use of Pulsed Electromagnetic Field Therapies." *Electromagnetic Biology and Medicine* 26 (3): 257–274.

Wunsch, A., and Matuschka, K. 2014. "A Controlled Trial to Determine the Efficacy of Red and Near-Infrared Light Treatment in Patient Satisfaction, Reduction of Fine Lines, Wrinkles, Skin Roughness, and Intradermal Collagen Density Increase." *Photomedicine and Laser Surgery* 32 (2): 93–100.

Chapter Twenty-Five

Balkwill, F., et al. 2001. "Role of Cytokines in Lymphatic Function and Regulation." *The Lancet* 357 (9259): 1221–1229.

Crinnion, W. J. 2011. "Sauna as a Valuable Clinical Tool for Cardiovascular, Autoimmune, and Toxicant-Associated Health Conditions." *Alternative Medicine Review* 16 (3): 215–225.

Heindel, J. J., and Blumberg, B. 2019. "Environmental Obesogens: Mechanisms and Controversies." *Annual Review of Pharmacology and Toxicology* 59: 89–106.

Klein, A. V., and Kiat, H. 2015. "Detox Diets for Toxin Elimination and Weight Management: A Critical Review of the Evidence." *Journal of Human Nutrition and Dietetics* 28 (6): 675–686.

Myers, S. P. 2004. "Detoxification Therapies: Core Concepts and Application in Naturopathic Medicine." *Journal of the Australian Traditional-Medicine Society* 10 (3): 112–117.

Rockson, S. G. 2001. "Lymphatic Transport of Macromolecules and Toxins." *Annual Review of Medicine* 52: 225–245.

Russo, E., et al. 2016. "Lymphatic System: An Integrated Interface for Immune Cell Trafficking and Antigen Presentation." *Seminars in Cell & Developmental Biology* 38: 28–34.

Szolnoky, G., et al. 2007. "Manual Lymph Drainage Reduces Oedema and Improves Quality of Life in Patients with Lipedema: A Prospective Study." *European Journal of Dermatology* 17 (2): 163–168.

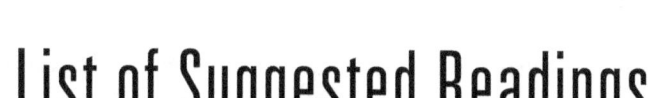

List of Suggested Readings

Non-Toxic: Guide to Living Healthy in a Chemical World by Aly Cohen, MD, and Frederick S. Vom Saal, PhD

The Hormone Reset Diet by Sara Gottfried, MD

The Hormone Cure by Sara Gottfried, MD

The Cortisol Connection by Shawn Talbott, PHD, FACSM

Eat for Health by Joel Fuhrman, MD

The Complete Anti-Inflammatory Diet for Beginners by Dorothy Calimeris and Lulu Cook

The Plant Paradox by Steve R. Gundry, MD

Medical Medium: Liver Rescue by Anthony William

Medical Medium: Secrets Behind Chronic and Mystery Illness and How to Finally Heal by Anthony William

Medical Medium: Cleanse to Heal by Anthony William

Food Sanity by Dr. David Friedman

Prescription for Herbal Living by Phyllis Balch, CNC

Prescription for Nutritional Healing by Phyllis Balch, CNC

The Complete Book of Ayurvedic Home Remedies by Vasant Lad, BAMS, MAS

Vibrational Medicine by Richard Gerber, MD

You are What You Think by David Stoop, MD

The Golden Key by Emmet Fox

How to Stop Worrying and Start Living by Dale Carnegie

Quick Reference Guide for Using Essential Oils by Connie and Alan Higley

Super Gut: A Four-Week Plan to Reprogram Your Microbiome by Dr. William Davis

Recommended Resources

- The Healthy Living app by the Environmental Working Group can be used to scan items and help search for clean products. Products that are EWG-verified have a score less than 7, are compliant with California Prop 65, and do not have EDC or cancer-causing ingredients. Or, visit www.ewg.org if you would rather go to the website instead of using the app.
- The Think Dirty-Shop Clean app also scans barcodes for ingredients.
- The Clearya app can alert you if a product has ingredients of concern. It works on Amazon and Walmart.com, but only if ingredients are listed.
- The site www.madesafe.org covers household items, personal care products, and more than EWG.
- The site www.thedetoxmarket.com allows you to try approved beauty products monthly.
- Visit www.endo-society.org for an updated consensus on EDCs.

- The site www.niehs.nih.gov is the National Institute of Environmental Health Sciences website for user-friendly information.
- The site https://chemtrust.org reports on efforts to reduce EDC exposure worldwide.
- For water testing, consider www.mytapscore.com which offers both in-lab and at-home comprehensive testing. Pace (www.pacelabs.com) can perform chemical and PFAS testing in several states. Please be sure that whichever company you choose is certified to do testing in your state.
- For laboratory screening for chemicals and toxins, consider Vibrant Wellness.
- To check for toxins in the water and air near you, go to www.scorecard.org to check what has been reported by your zip code.

Acknowledgments

I would like to take this special moment to give thanks to God who has guided me toward this newfound knowledge and inspired me to share this with all of you. I thank my loving husband, Andre, for his love, patience, and steadfast faith in me throughout this entire endeavor. Many thanks to my parents, Jacques and Yvette, for their love, encouragement, and prayers over all my life's challenges. My heartfelt thanks to my brother Jacques Jr., my sister-in-law Ramona, my brother's children Alex and JP, my best friend Nadine, and my numerous family and friends who have shown their love and support for me. I am so blessed to have worked with my life coaches, Dr. Maiysha Clairborne and Dr. Catherine Woodhouse, who enabled me to free myself from the mental barriers blocking me from making this huge step. I am grateful for the guidance and instructions given by the Goldberg Tener Clinic which devised a personalized plan to reverse the chronic inflammation and diseases that had been plaguing me. Finally, much appreciation goes to environmental toxin expert Lara Adler whose very thorough and informative course, "Talking Toxins," equipped me with the knowledge to grow and advocate for change regarding this growing threat to us all.

About the Author

Dr. S. M. René, The EDC Doc,™ is an experienced board-certified endocrinologist who has been practicing for the past twenty-five years. Dr. René earned a medical degree at Howard University in Washington, DC. Internship and residency in internal medicine were completed at the Mayo Clinic in Jacksonville, Florida, followed by fellowship training in endocrinology and metabolism at Emory University in Atlanta, Georgia. Dr. René was awarded the prestigious honor of Fellow of the American Association of Clinical Endocrinology for achievements in the field of endocrinology. Dr. René has done numerous regional speaking engagements for various pharmaceutical companies addressing topics relating to hypothyroidism, diabetes, and metabolic syndrome. Medical expertise includes performing thyroid biopsies, PCOS, thyroid cancer, and general endocrine disorders. Distinctions awarded include the Top Doctors of America in Endocrinology from 2017 to 2024, Best in Georgia in Endocrinology recognition in 2024 and 2025, and the Continental Who's Who recognition in 2017 and 2024. As Dr. René says, "The most integral key to my success is a steadfast faith in God, coupled with the unwavering support from my spouse, family, and friends."

www.ingramcontent.com/pod-product-compliance
Lightning Source LLC
Chambersburg PA
CBHW020453030426
42337CB00011B/100